Fatty Liver Diet Recipes

Recipes for Reversing Fatty Liver and Living Your Healthiest Life

Dr. Ava Montgomery

© Copyright 2024 by Dr. Ava Montgomery - All rights reserved.

Table of Contents

Introduction 3

Chapter 1: Understanding Fatty Liver Disease
The Root Causes and How It Impacts Your Health 7

Chapter 2: The Science of Reversing Fatty Liver
What Works and What Doesn't 63

Chapter 3: The Ideal Fatty Liver Diet
A 7-Day Meal Plan to Get You Started 89

Chapter 4: 100+ Delicious Fatty Liver-Friendly Recipes for Every Meal of the Day 119

Chapter 5: Meal Prep Mastery for Fatty Liver Disease
Make Your Week Easy 165

Chapter 6: Understanding Liver Detox
What Your Liver Really Needs 193

Chapter 7: Exercise for Liver Health
Best Practices for Fatty Liver Reversal 223

Chapter 8: Managing Stress and Emotional Health
A Key Component in Reversing Fatty Liver 250

Chapter 9: Building Long-Term
Habits for Healthy Liver Function 277

Chapter 10: Expert Interviews from Leading Doctors, Nutritionists, and Researchers 304

Conclusion 331

References 333

Author Name: Dr. Ava Montgomery 335

Disclaimer 337

Copyright 338

Legal Notice 339

Introduction

Reversing Fatty Liver for a Healthier, Happier Life

Welcome to *Fatty Liver Diet Recipes: 100+ Recipes for Reversing Fatty Liver and Living Your Healthiest Life*. Whether you've recently been diagnosed with fatty liver disease, are already aware of its potential dangers, or are simply looking to improve your liver health and overall well-being, this book is designed to guide you every step of the way. Through a combination of scientifically-backed information, delicious and easy-to-make recipes, and holistic lifestyle strategies, you will find everything you need to reclaim your health and reverse fatty liver disease naturally.

What is Fatty Liver Disease?

Fatty liver disease occurs when there is an excessive buildup of fat in your liver cells. While a small amount of fat in the liver is normal, too much can interfere with the liver's ability to function properly. Over time, fatty liver can progress into more severe conditions such as Non-Alcoholic Steatohepatitis (NASH) or cirrhosis, both of which can be life-threatening if left untreated. The good news is that fatty liver disease is often reversible, especially in its early stages. The key to reversing fatty liver is not just medical intervention, but also making the right dietary and lifestyle choices—something you can take control of today.

The Power of Nutrition and Lifestyle

At the heart of reversing fatty liver is the power of nutrition. While medications and medical treatments are essential, what you put into your body every day can play an even more significant role in your liver's healing process. This book is built on the understanding that food is medicine, and by nourishing your body with the right nutrients, you can help restore your liver to health.

In the following pages, you'll discover the importance of choosing foods that are rich in antioxidants, anti-inflammatory compounds, and essential nutrients that support liver function. You'll also learn how to manage blood sugar levels, reduce inflammation, and detoxify your liver naturally—all through the foods you eat. This is not a fad diet, but a sustainable, long-term approach to improving your liver health and living a vibrant life.

Your Journey Starts Here

In this book, we don't just give you recipes—we give you the tools and knowledge to change your life. Each chapter is designed to empower you with actionable information, including:

- **A complete understanding of fatty liver disease**: You'll gain insight into the root causes, risk factors, and how fatty liver disease progresses.
- **A step-by-step guide to reversing fatty liver**: From the science behind liver health to practical strategies for success, we provide you with the knowledge you need to reclaim your health.
- **100+ liver-friendly recipes**: These carefully crafted recipes are designed to be not only delicious but also

healing for your liver. Whether you're making a simple breakfast, a hearty lunch, or a nourishing dinner, you'll have access to a wide variety of meals that support liver detox, reduce fat accumulation, and promote overall wellness.
- **Meal prep strategies**: Learn how to make your healthy liver meals easy and convenient, with step-by-step meal prep techniques that save you time and effort.

Beyond just recipes, we will explore lifestyle changes that support liver health—such as regular exercise, stress management, quality sleep, and building sustainable habits. By combining good food with a holistic approach to health, you can reverse the damage done to your liver and take control of your overall well-being.

What Makes This Book Different?

There are many books out there on fatty liver disease, but what sets this one apart is our holistic, practical approach. Many books simply offer recipes or a general overview of liver health, but here, you'll find a complete resource that guides you through every aspect of fatty liver management. From understanding the disease to building lifelong habits, this book is your go-to guide for reversing fatty liver in a way that's both effective and sustainable.

We take a compassionate, patient-centered approach because we understand that every journey is unique. Whether you're just beginning or are already on the path to liver recovery, this book is designed to meet you where you are and provide you with the tools you need to succeed.

A Healthier Future Awaits

Reversing fatty liver disease is not a quick fix—it's a lifestyle change, but one that will benefit you for years to come. By following the steps outlined in this book, you'll not only be supporting your liver but also improving your overall health, boosting your energy, and living a more vibrant, fulfilling life.

As you begin this journey, remember that small changes can have a big impact. Every healthy meal, every mindful decision to prioritize your health, and every new habit you embrace brings you closer to the healthiest version of yourself. Your liver—and your life—will thank you for it.

Let's get started on the path to a healthier liver and a happier, more energetic you.

Welcome to your new, liver-healthy life.

Chapter 1: Understanding Fatty Liver Disease – The Root Causes and How It Impacts Your Health

Fatty liver disease is becoming increasingly common worldwide, and understanding its root causes is the first step toward managing and reversing it. In this chapter, we will explore what fatty liver disease is, how it develops, and its potential long-term impacts on your health. We'll also examine the key factors that contribute to its onset, so you can make informed choices in reversing or preventing its progression.

What is Fatty Liver Disease?

Fatty liver disease (FLD) occurs when excess fat builds up in the liver cells. The liver is essential for many vital functions, including detoxifying the body, producing proteins, and storing energy. Under normal conditions, the liver contains small amounts of fat. However, when fat exceeds 5% to 10% of the liver's total weight, it can disrupt liver function and lead to fatty liver disease.

There are two primary forms of fatty liver disease:

1. **Non-Alcoholic Fatty Liver Disease (NAFLD)**: This is the most common form and occurs in people who do not drink alcohol or consume it in excess. NAFLD can range from simple fat accumulation in the liver to a more serious condition known as non-alcoholic steatohepatitis (NASH).
2. **Alcoholic Fatty Liver Disease (AFLD)**: This form of fatty liver disease is caused by heavy alcohol consumption. When the liver processes alcohol, it

produces toxins that can damage liver cells, leading to fat buildup and inflammation.

NAFLD is particularly concerning because it is often asymptomatic, meaning people can live with the condition for years without realizing it. Left unchecked, fatty liver disease can progress into more severe liver conditions, including cirrhosis, liver failure, and liver cancer.

The Stages of Fatty Liver Disease

Fatty liver disease develops in stages, and understanding these stages helps to explain how the disease progresses if left untreated:

1. **Simple Fatty Liver (Steatosis)**: In the earliest stage of NAFLD, fat accumulates in the liver cells without causing significant inflammation or damage. At this stage, the liver is still functioning normally, and most people experience no symptoms. While it may seem harmless, simple steatosis can eventually progress if not managed through diet and lifestyle changes.
2. **Non-Alcoholic Steatohepatitis (NASH)**: In this more advanced stage, the accumulation of fat in the liver is accompanied by inflammation and liver cell damage. NASH increases the risk of fibrosis, a condition where scar tissue forms in the liver. If left untreated, NASH can lead to cirrhosis or liver failure.
3. **Cirrhosis**: This is the final stage of fatty liver disease, characterized by significant scarring of the liver. As cirrhosis progresses, the liver loses its ability to function properly, leading to complications such as liver cancer, gastrointestinal bleeding, and ascites (fluid

buildup in the abdomen). Cirrhosis is often irreversible, and a liver transplant may be required in severe cases.

How Fatty Liver Disease Develops: The Root Causes

Fatty liver disease doesn't happen overnight. It is the result of a complex interaction between various genetic, lifestyle, and environmental factors. Understanding the key drivers of fatty liver disease can help you make informed choices to prevent or reverse it.

1. **Poor Diet**: A diet high in processed foods, refined sugars, and unhealthy fats (particularly trans fats) can contribute to the accumulation of fat in the liver. Diets rich in fructose, found in sugary beverages and processed snacks, are particularly harmful. Consuming more calories than the body needs leads to fat storage, some of which may accumulate in the liver.
2. **Obesity and Overweight**: One of the biggest risk factors for fatty liver disease is obesity. Excess body fat, particularly around the abdominal area, increases the liver's fat content. The liver, tasked with metabolizing fat, begins to store excess fat, leading to fatty liver. The risk is particularly high in people who are obese and have abdominal fat accumulation.
3. **Insulin Resistance and Type 2 Diabetes**: Insulin resistance, a hallmark of type 2 diabetes, is closely linked to fatty liver disease. When the body becomes resistant to insulin, blood sugar levels rise, and the liver starts producing more fat. Insulin resistance is a key driver of both NAFLD and NASH, as the liver cells begin to store excess fat in response to increased blood sugar levels.

4. **High Cholesterol and Triglycerides**: Elevated cholesterol levels and high triglycerides, often seen in individuals with metabolic syndrome, increase the risk of fatty liver disease. These conditions result in the liver being overwhelmed with lipids, leading to fat accumulation.
5. **Genetic Factors**: While lifestyle factors play a significant role in the development of fatty liver disease, genetics can also influence an individual's susceptibility. Studies have identified certain genes that can make individuals more prone to developing NAFLD, even if they maintain a healthy weight or eat a relatively balanced diet.
6. **Other Health Conditions**: Several other health conditions are linked to fatty liver disease, including high blood pressure, polycystic ovary syndrome (PCOS), sleep apnea, and hypothyroidism. Inflammatory conditions like autoimmune hepatitis and viral infections such as hepatitis C can also damage the liver and contribute to the development of fatty liver disease.
7. **Alcohol Consumption**: Excessive alcohol consumption is a major cause of alcoholic fatty liver disease. The liver metabolizes alcohol, and when consumed in large quantities, alcohol disrupts the liver's ability to function normally, causing fat to accumulate in liver cells.

How Fatty Liver Disease Impacts Your Health

Fatty liver disease may seem like a silent condition at first, but over time, it can have far-reaching consequences for your overall health. Here's how it can affect your body:

1. **Metabolic Disruption**: Fatty liver disease is closely linked to metabolic dysfunction. Individuals with NAFLD are more likely to develop insulin resistance, high blood pressure, and type 2 diabetes. The liver plays a key role in regulating metabolism, so when it's not functioning optimally, it can lead to a cascade of metabolic disturbances.
2. **Increased Risk of Heart Disease**: Research has shown that fatty liver disease increases the risk of cardiovascular diseases, including heart attack and stroke. The same risk factors that contribute to fatty liver disease—such as high cholesterol, obesity, and insulin resistance—are also risk factors for heart disease.
3. **Chronic Inflammation**: As fatty liver disease progresses to NASH, the liver becomes inflamed. Chronic inflammation in the liver can cause long-term damage, including fibrosis and cirrhosis. Inflammation is also a systemic issue, potentially affecting other organs and tissues, contributing to conditions like arthritis, kidney disease, and even certain cancers.
4. **Liver Damage and Scarring**: When left untreated, fatty liver disease leads to liver damage and scarring (fibrosis), impairing the liver's ability to detoxify the body, store nutrients, and regulate blood sugar. In severe cases, cirrhosis may develop, leading to liver failure and the need for a transplant.
5. **Impact on Mental Health**: People with fatty liver disease may experience an increased risk of depression and anxiety. The link between liver health and mental well-being is complex, as the liver is responsible for metabolizing toxins, and liver dysfunction can result in

the accumulation of harmful substances that affect brain function.

What This Means for You

Fatty liver disease is a progressive condition that can severely affect your health if left unaddressed. The good news is that, in most cases, fatty liver disease can be reversed, especially in its early stages. By understanding its root causes, you can take proactive steps to reverse the damage and improve your liver health. With the right diet, lifestyle changes, and proper care, you can manage fatty liver disease and reduce your risk of more serious complications, leading to a healthier, longer life.

In the next chapters, we'll explore the specific dietary strategies, meal plans, and lifestyle modifications that can help you reverse fatty liver disease and protect your liver for the long term.

What is Fatty Liver Disease?

Fatty liver disease is a condition in which excess fat accumulates in the liver cells. While the liver naturally contains a small amount of fat, an excess can impair its ability to function properly. This buildup of fat is often a silent process, developing gradually over time, with minimal or no symptoms in its early stages. Despite its seemingly benign onset, fatty liver disease can lead to serious health problems if left untreated, ranging from inflammation and scarring of the liver to cirrhosis and liver failure.

In this section, we'll dive deeper into what fatty liver disease is, how it develops, and why it's critical to address it early. Understanding this condition is the first step in reversing its effects and improving your liver health.

The Liver's Role in Your Health

Before we delve into fatty liver disease, it's essential to understand the vital functions the liver performs. The liver is the body's largest internal organ and is responsible for more than 500 essential functions, including:

- **Detoxification**: The liver helps filter toxins from the blood, including waste products from medications, alcohol, and harmful chemicals.
- **Metabolism**: It converts nutrients from food into substances that the body can use, including storing glucose as glycogen, and synthesizing cholesterol and proteins.
- **Digestive Aid**: The liver produces bile, which is crucial for digesting fats and absorbing fat-soluble vitamins (A, D, E, and K).
- **Blood Clotting**: The liver produces proteins that help the blood clot properly and prevent excessive bleeding.

When the liver is healthy, it performs these functions efficiently. However, when fat accumulates within the liver, it can disrupt these processes, leading to potential health problems.

Types of Fatty Liver Disease

There are two main types of fatty liver disease: **Non-Alcoholic Fatty Liver Disease (NAFLD)** and **Alcoholic Fatty Liver Disease (AFLD)**. Although they share similar characteristics, they have different causes and risk factors.

1. Non-Alcoholic Fatty Liver Disease (NAFLD)

NAFLD is the most common form of fatty liver disease, accounting for approximately 75% of cases. As the name suggests, this condition occurs in people who do not drink alcohol or only consume it in moderation. NAFLD is typically associated with metabolic risk factors such as obesity, type 2 diabetes, and high cholesterol, and is often seen in people who are overweight or obese.

NAFLD encompasses a range of liver abnormalities, from simple fat accumulation (steatosis) to more severe forms of liver damage. The key characteristic of NAFLD is the buildup of fat in the liver cells without significant inflammation or liver damage.

2. Alcoholic Fatty Liver Disease (AFLD)

AFLD, on the other hand, is caused by excessive alcohol consumption. Alcohol is metabolized by the liver, and when consumed in large quantities, it can overwhelm the liver's ability to process it. This leads to fat accumulation within liver cells, which can eventually lead to inflammation, scarring, and liver damage. AFLD typically occurs in people who consume large amounts of alcohol over an extended period.

In both NAFLD and AFLD, fat buildup in the liver is often asymptomatic in the early stages, making the disease difficult to detect without proper screening.

How Does Fatty Liver Disease Develop?

Fatty liver disease develops when the body accumulates more fat in the liver than it can process and eliminate. This can happen for several reasons, including poor diet, sedentary lifestyle, or genetic factors. To understand how the liver becomes fatty, we need to look at what's happening at the cellular level.

1. **Fat Metabolism in the Liver**

   The liver plays a central role in fat metabolism. When the body consumes more calories than it needs, excess energy is stored in fat cells. Some of this fat is transferred to the liver, where it can either be processed and used for energy or stored for later use. Under normal circumstances, the liver can handle this process efficiently, and the fat is metabolized in a balanced way.

2. **Disruption of Fat Processing**

   However, when the liver becomes overwhelmed with fat—due to poor diet, obesity, insulin resistance, or excessive alcohol consumption—it may struggle to process the fat efficiently. The fat accumulates in the liver cells, and the liver can no longer process it in the usual manner. This leads to the formation of fat droplets within liver cells, which can cause liver inflammation and damage if left unchecked.

3. **The Role of Insulin Resistance**

   One of the primary contributors to fatty liver disease is insulin resistance, a condition in which the body becomes less responsive to insulin. Insulin is a hormone that helps regulate blood sugar levels and fat storage. When insulin resistance occurs, the liver becomes less effective at clearing glucose from the bloodstream and more prone to storing excess fat. This creates a cycle where fat accumulates in the liver, which worsens insulin resistance and leads to further fat storage.

4. **Oxidative Stress and Inflammation**

   Over time, fat accumulation in the liver can trigger oxidative stress and inflammation. As fat builds up, it can lead to the release of reactive oxygen species (ROS) that damage liver cells. This damage prompts an inflammatory response that can further impair liver function. When inflammation becomes chronic, it can lead to fibrosis (the formation of scar tissue) and, in severe cases, cirrhosis.

Symptoms and Diagnosis

Fatty liver disease is often called a "silent" condition because it typically doesn't cause noticeable symptoms in the early stages. In fact, many people with fatty liver disease don't realize they have it until they undergo routine blood tests or imaging studies. However, as the condition progresses, more noticeable symptoms may appear, including:

- Fatigue or low energy levels
- Unexplained weight loss or difficulty losing weight
- Abdominal discomfort or a feeling of fullness in the upper right side of the abdomen
- Jaundice (yellowing of the skin or eyes) in severe cases
- Swelling or fluid buildup in the abdomen (ascites)

Diagnosing fatty liver disease typically involves a combination of:

- **Blood tests** to check liver enzyme levels (elevated liver enzymes can indicate liver inflammation).
- **Imaging tests** such as ultrasound, CT scans, or MRI to detect fat accumulation in the liver.
- **Liver biopsy** (in some cases) to assess the severity of liver damage and determine whether the condition has progressed to NASH or cirrhosis.

Risk Factors for Fatty Liver Disease

Several factors can increase the risk of developing fatty liver disease. These include:

- **Obesity**: Excess body weight, especially abdominal fat, is a significant risk factor for fatty liver disease.
- **Diabetes and Insulin Resistance**: People with type 2 diabetes or those with prediabetes are at a higher risk due to insulin resistance.

- **High Cholesterol and Triglycerides**: Elevated levels of cholesterol and triglycerides in the blood can contribute to fat buildup in the liver.
- **Poor Diet**: Diets high in refined sugars, processed foods, and unhealthy fats can increase fat accumulation in the liver.
- **Alcohol Consumption**: Heavy or long-term alcohol use is a leading cause of fatty liver disease.
- **Genetics**: Family history can increase the likelihood of developing fatty liver disease.
- **Age and Gender**: People over the age of 50 and postmenopausal women are at higher risk.

Why Fatty Liver Disease Matters

While fatty liver disease may not show immediate symptoms, it can have serious long-term health consequences if left untreated. Over time, fat accumulation in the liver can lead to liver inflammation, fibrosis, cirrhosis, and eventually liver failure. Additionally, fatty liver disease is linked to an increased risk of heart disease, stroke, and other metabolic conditions like type 2 diabetes and hypertension.

The good news is that fatty liver disease is reversible, especially in its early stages. Through diet, exercise, and lifestyle changes, it's possible to reduce liver fat, reverse inflammation, and prevent further liver damage.

Next Steps

Understanding what fatty liver disease is and how it develops is just the first step. In the following chapters, we will discuss the causes and risk factors in more detail, as well as provide actionable strategies and recipes that will help you reverse fatty liver disease and improve your liver health for the long term.

By taking control of your diet and lifestyle, you can begin to repair your liver, reduce fat accumulation, and ultimately restore your health.

Exploring the Different Stages of Fatty Liver Disease: NAFLD and NASH

Fatty liver disease is not a single, static condition. It progresses through different stages, ranging from simple fat accumulation in the liver to more severe forms of liver damage, potentially leading to liver failure. The progression of fatty liver disease is often subtle, and many individuals may not be aware of its development until it reaches a critical stage. Understanding these stages—particularly **Non-Alcoholic Fatty Liver Disease (NAFLD)** and **Non-Alcoholic Steatohepatitis (NASH)**—is crucial for early intervention and management.

In this section, we will explore the different stages of fatty liver disease, focusing on NAFLD and NASH, and how they affect your liver health.

1. Non-Alcoholic Fatty Liver Disease (NAFLD)

NAFLD is the earliest stage of fatty liver disease and is characterized by the accumulation of excess fat in the liver cells. As the name suggests, this condition occurs in individuals who do not consume alcohol or consume it in moderation, making it distinct from alcoholic fatty liver disease. NAFLD is often referred to as a "silent" condition because it typically doesn't cause noticeable symptoms in its early stages, which makes it difficult to detect without proper medical screening.

How NAFLD Develops:

In NAFLD, the liver cells store excess fat, but there is no significant inflammation or damage to liver tissue. This fat accumulation can result from several factors, including:

- **Obesity**: One of the most common causes of NAFLD, especially excess visceral (abdominal) fat.
- **Insulin Resistance**: A hallmark of type 2 diabetes and metabolic syndrome, insulin resistance prevents the body from properly managing glucose and fat, contributing to fat storage in the liver.
- **Poor Diet**: Diets high in processed foods, sugar, and unhealthy fats can lead to fat buildup in the liver.
- **Sedentary Lifestyle**: Lack of physical activity can lead to weight gain and insulin resistance, both of which are major contributors to NAFLD.
- **Genetic Factors**: A family history of fatty liver disease can increase the risk of developing NAFLD.

At this stage, the liver is still functioning normally, and liver enzymes (such as ALT and AST) may be in the normal range. Although NAFLD can remain undiagnosed for years, early detection through imaging (such as ultrasound or MRI) or blood tests is possible, especially in those with risk factors.

Prognosis of NAFLD:

NAFLD is often considered a benign condition in its early stages, but it can progress over time if the underlying causes (such as obesity or insulin resistance) are not addressed. The good news is that **NAFLD is reversible**, especially with lifestyle changes like improved diet, regular exercise, and weight management.

2. Non-Alcoholic Steatohepatitis (NASH)

NASH is the more advanced and concerning stage of fatty liver disease. It occurs when the fat accumulation in the liver leads to **inflammation** and **liver cell damage**, which can cause liver scarring (fibrosis). NASH is considered a more severe form of NAFLD and can lead to further liver complications, including cirrhosis, liver cancer, and liver failure.

How NASH Develops:

NASH develops when fat buildup in the liver causes an inflammatory response. This inflammation can damage liver cells, leading to scarring, or fibrosis. The process typically begins after a prolonged period of fat accumulation in the liver, often in individuals who have long-standing obesity, diabetes, or metabolic syndrome.

Several factors contribute to the progression from NAFLD to NASH:

- **Oxidative Stress**: The liver fat, when metabolized, can produce free radicals (reactive oxygen species or ROS)

that damage liver cells. This oxidative stress triggers an inflammatory response that accelerates liver damage.
- **Inflammation**: Chronic low-grade inflammation is a hallmark of NASH. The body's immune system sends white blood cells to the liver to repair damage, but these cells can worsen the inflammation and injury to the liver.
- **Fatty Acid Toxicity**: Excessive fat in the liver can cause toxic effects, especially in the presence of insulin resistance. The liver becomes overwhelmed by the fat it cannot process, leading to further damage.
- **Fibrosis Formation**: As the inflammation persists, the liver begins to repair itself by producing fibrous tissue. This scarring is referred to as fibrosis, and the severity of fibrosis can range from mild to severe.

Symptoms of NASH:

Unlike NAFLD, NASH can cause noticeable symptoms, including:

- **Fatigue**: Persistent tiredness, often unrelated to sleep quality or quantity.
- **Abdominal Discomfort**: Pain or a feeling of fullness in the upper right side of the abdomen, where the liver is located.
- **Weight Loss**: Unexplained weight loss or difficulty maintaining a healthy weight.
- **Jaundice**: A yellowing of the skin and eyes, which is a sign of liver dysfunction.
- **Swelling**: Fluid retention in the abdomen (ascites) or legs.

While the symptoms may be mild at first, if NASH progresses without treatment, it can lead to serious liver complications.

Diagnosis of NASH:

Diagnosing NASH can be challenging, as many of the symptoms overlap with other conditions. Doctors often use a combination of blood tests, imaging studies (like ultrasound or elastography), and sometimes a liver biopsy to confirm the presence of NASH and assess the extent of liver damage. A liver biopsy is the gold standard for diagnosing NASH, as it allows for the direct assessment of liver inflammation and fibrosis.

Prognosis of NASH:

Unlike NAFLD, NASH can lead to progressive liver damage. If left untreated, the inflammation and fibrosis caused by NASH can lead to the following:

- **Cirrhosis**: A severe form of liver scarring that can impair liver function and lead to liver failure.
- **Liver Cancer**: NASH is a known risk factor for hepatocellular carcinoma (HCC), a form of liver cancer.
- **Liver Failure**: As the liver becomes increasingly damaged, it can lose its ability to function, leading to a condition known as liver failure.

The progression from NASH to cirrhosis and liver cancer typically occurs over several years or even decades, making early intervention critical. However, NASH is a treatable condition, especially in the earlier stages, with appropriate dietary and lifestyle changes.

3. The Progression of Fatty Liver Disease: NAFLD to NASH to Cirrhosis

Fatty liver disease progresses through stages, and understanding this progression is essential for preventing further liver damage:

- **Stage 1 – NAFLD (Non-Alcoholic Fatty Liver Disease)**: Fat accumulates in the liver cells without causing significant inflammation or damage. Liver function remains normal.
- **Stage 2 – NASH (Non-Alcoholic Steatohepatitis)**: Fat accumulation in the liver triggers inflammation and liver cell damage, leading to scarring (fibrosis).
- **Stage 3 – Fibrosis**: The liver begins to develop significant scarring due to chronic inflammation. Liver function may start to decline.
- **Stage 4 – Cirrhosis**: The liver becomes severely scarred, losing its ability to function properly. Cirrhosis is a life-threatening condition that can lead to liver failure, complications like varices (enlarged blood vessels), and liver cancer.

In the early stages (NAFLD and NASH), fatty liver disease is reversible with lifestyle changes, but once cirrhosis sets in, the damage is permanent and can lead to life-threatening complications. Early detection and intervention are key to preventing the progression of the disease.

4. Reversing NAFLD and NASH

While fatty liver disease can progress to severe stages if left unchecked, the good news is that both NAFLD and NASH are

reversible in their early stages. The primary treatment is focused on addressing the underlying causes, such as:

- **Weight loss**: Gradual weight loss through a healthy diet and regular exercise can significantly reduce liver fat.
- **Improving Insulin Sensitivity**: Managing diabetes, improving blood sugar control, and reducing insulin resistance can help prevent further fat buildup in the liver.
- **Dietary Changes**: A balanced diet, low in processed sugars and unhealthy fats, can help reduce liver fat and inflammation.
- **Avoiding Alcohol**: For those with NASH, avoiding alcohol is crucial in preventing further liver damage.

The Science Behind Liver Function and How Fatty Liver Disrupts It

The liver is a vital organ that plays a central role in maintaining overall health. It is the body's primary detoxifier, energy producer, and regulator of many biochemical processes. Understanding the science behind liver function and how fatty liver disease disrupts it is key to appreciating why the condition can have such a significant impact on your health.

In this section, we will explore the intricate mechanisms of liver function, how it contributes to your body's well-being, and the way fatty liver disease impairs these critical functions.

1. The Essential Functions of the Liver

The liver is one of the most hardworking organs in your body, responsible for performing hundreds of essential tasks. Here are some of the most important functions it performs:

a) Metabolism and Energy Regulation

- **Glucose Storage and Release**: The liver helps regulate blood sugar levels by storing excess glucose as glycogen after meals. Between meals, it releases glucose into the bloodstream to maintain a stable energy supply, a process known as **gluconeogenesis**.
- **Fat Metabolism**: The liver is responsible for breaking down fats into fatty acids and cholesterol. It also synthesizes proteins necessary for fat metabolism, such as lipoproteins.
- **Protein Synthesis**: The liver produces proteins essential for many bodily functions, including blood clotting (e.g., fibrinogen), albumin (which helps maintain blood volume), and enzymes involved in digestion.

b) Detoxification and Waste Removal

- **Filtering Toxins**: One of the liver's most vital roles is detoxifying harmful substances from the blood. It breaks down drugs, alcohol, and environmental toxins, rendering them less harmful or ready for excretion via the kidneys or intestines.
- **Ammonia Detoxification**: The liver converts ammonia, a byproduct of protein metabolism, into urea, which is then excreted in the urine. Without this function, toxic

ammonia would build up in the blood, leading to potentially fatal complications.

c) Bile Production and Digestion

- **Bile Production**: The liver produces bile, a digestive fluid that is stored in the gallbladder and released into the intestines during digestion. Bile is crucial for the breakdown and absorption of dietary fats and fat-soluble vitamins (A, D, E, K).
- **Cholesterol Management**: The liver helps regulate blood cholesterol levels by converting excess cholesterol into bile acids, which are then excreted.

d) Immune System Regulation

- **Immunity**: The liver contains a large number of immune cells, including Kupffer cells, which help fight infections and clear bacteria from the bloodstream. It also plays a role in producing proteins involved in inflammation and the immune response.

2. How Fatty Liver Disease Disrupts Liver Function

Fatty liver disease, particularly in its early stages, may not cause significant symptoms. However, as the condition progresses, it impairs the liver's ability to perform its critical functions effectively. Here's how fatty liver disease disrupts liver health:

a) Disruption of Fat Metabolism

- **Fat Buildup**: In a healthy liver, fat is metabolized and used for energy or stored in a regulated manner. However, in fatty liver disease (both NAFLD and NASH), excess fat accumulates in the liver cells. This excess fat interferes with the liver's ability to metabolize and manage fatty acids, leading to further fat storage and, eventually, liver inflammation.
- **Insulin Resistance**: A primary cause of fatty liver disease is insulin resistance, where the body's cells do not respond effectively to insulin. As a result, the liver produces more glucose and stores more fat. Insulin resistance exacerbates fat buildup, further disrupting metabolic processes in the liver.

b) Inflammation and Liver Cell Damage (NASH)

- **Inflammation**: In NASH, fat accumulation in liver cells triggers an inflammatory response. This inflammation leads to the release of cytokines and other molecules that cause liver cell damage. The inflammation also impairs the liver's ability to produce proteins and enzymes necessary for metabolism.
- **Liver Fibrosis**: Chronic inflammation in the liver leads to the formation of scar tissue, a process known as fibrosis. As fibrosis advances, the liver becomes stiffer, and its normal function becomes impaired. Fibrosis can also restrict blood flow within the liver, further disrupting its ability to perform metabolic functions.
- **Oxidative Stress**: The excess fat in the liver generates reactive oxygen species (ROS), which cause oxidative stress. This damages liver cells and accelerates

inflammation, contributing to the progression from simple fatty liver (NAFLD) to NASH, and eventually cirrhosis.

c) Impaired Detoxification

- **Toxin Accumulation**: When the liver is overwhelmed by excess fat and inflammation, its ability to filter toxins and harmful substances decreases. This can lead to a buildup of toxins in the body, further harming liver cells and other organs.
- **Ammonia Build-up**: As fatty liver disease progresses, the liver's capacity to process ammonia diminishes. This can lead to an increase in ammonia levels in the bloodstream, causing a condition known as **hepatic encephalopathy**, which can lead to confusion, altered mental states, and in severe cases, coma.

d) Impaired Bile Production and Digestion

- **Disruption in Bile Secretion**: Fatty liver disease, particularly in advanced stages, can hinder the liver's ability to produce and secrete bile. This leads to impaired digestion, particularly the breakdown and absorption of dietary fats and fat-soluble vitamins (A, D, E, K).
- **Gallstones**: Since bile production is impacted, fatty liver disease may increase the risk of developing gallstones, as bile is not processed or secreted efficiently, leading to an imbalance in bile components.

e) Impaired Immune Function

- **Impaired Immune Response**: As the liver becomes increasingly damaged, its ability to filter harmful microorganisms and regulate immune responses weakens. This can result in increased susceptibility to infections and reduced ability to heal from injury.
- **Chronic Inflammation**: The inflammation seen in NASH not only damages liver cells but can also alter the liver's immune response, contributing to a cycle of chronic inflammation that worsens liver damage over time.

3. The Progressive Nature of Fatty Liver Disease

In the early stages of fatty liver disease (NAFLD), the liver's function may not be significantly impacted, and liver cells can recover if the underlying causes (such as obesity, poor diet, or insulin resistance) are addressed. However, as fatty liver progresses to NASH and fibrosis, liver function becomes increasingly compromised:

- **NAFLD**: While the liver still performs most of its functions, excess fat accumulation can hinder its efficiency. The liver may struggle to regulate blood sugar, produce proteins, or break down fat effectively.
- **NASH**: In addition to fat accumulation, liver inflammation and fibrosis begin to impair essential functions. Toxin processing becomes less efficient, and bile production is reduced.
- **Cirrhosis**: As the liver becomes severely scarred, many functions are lost entirely. The liver's ability to detoxify

the body, regulate metabolism, and produce necessary proteins becomes severely compromised.

4. How Reversing Fatty Liver Disease Can Restore Liver Function

Fortunately, early stages of fatty liver disease are reversible, and with the right interventions, many of the liver's disrupted functions can be restored. The key lies in addressing the root causes:

- **Diet**: A balanced, liver-friendly diet rich in antioxidants, healthy fats, and fiber can reduce fat accumulation and inflammation in the liver. A low-sugar, low-refined-carbohydrate diet helps improve insulin sensitivity.
- **Exercise**: Regular physical activity helps reduce liver fat, improve insulin sensitivity, and reduce systemic inflammation, aiding in the restoration of liver function.
- **Weight Loss**: Gradual weight loss through a healthy lifestyle can reduce liver fat, reverse insulin resistance, and reduce the risk of progressing to NASH or cirrhosis.
- **Avoiding Alcohol**: Limiting or eliminating alcohol consumption prevents additional strain on the liver and allows it to heal.

Risk Factors and Common Misconceptions About Fatty Liver Disease

Fatty liver disease, particularly Non-Alcoholic Fatty Liver Disease (NAFLD) and its more severe form, Non-Alcoholic Steatohepatitis (NASH), is a growing health concern globally. While many people may not even realize they have fatty liver disease, it's crucial to understand the risk factors that contribute to its development and progression. Equally important are the common misconceptions that can prevent effective management and prevention. In this chapter, we will dive into the key risk factors and debunk some myths surrounding fatty liver disease to provide a clearer, more accurate picture of this condition.

1. Risk Factors for Fatty Liver Disease

Fatty liver disease can affect anyone, but certain lifestyle factors, genetic predispositions, and underlying health conditions make some people more susceptible. Understanding these risk factors is the first step toward preventing and managing the condition.

a) Obesity and Excess Body Fat

- **Abdominal Fat**: One of the most significant risk factors for fatty liver disease is obesity, particularly the accumulation of visceral fat around the abdomen. Visceral fat surrounds the internal organs and is metabolically active, releasing fatty acids and inflammatory signals that can damage the liver.
- **Insulin Resistance**: Obesity, particularly when associated with excess abdominal fat, contributes to insulin resistance. As the body's cells become less responsive to insulin, the liver starts to accumulate more fat and becomes less efficient in its normal metabolic functions.

b) Poor Diet and Nutritional Deficiencies

- **High Sugar and Refined Carbohydrates**: Diets rich in sugar, refined carbohydrates (such as white bread and pastries), and sugary beverages (including sodas) are key contributors to the development of fatty liver disease. Excessive sugar intake leads to insulin resistance and increased fat storage in the liver.
- **Trans Fats and Processed Foods**: Diets high in unhealthy fats, such as trans fats found in processed foods, contribute to inflammation and fat accumulation in the liver. These fats are harder for the body to metabolize, which can lead to a buildup of fat within liver cells.
- **Nutrient Imbalance**: Deficiencies in essential nutrients like antioxidants (vitamin E, C) and omega-3 fatty acids can hinder the liver's ability to repair itself, increasing the risk of liver damage.

c) Type 2 Diabetes and Insulin Resistance

- **Insulin Resistance**: Type 2 diabetes is strongly associated with fatty liver disease because insulin resistance is a primary cause of fat buildup in the liver. When insulin doesn't work properly, glucose levels in the bloodstream rise, and the liver responds by storing more fat.
- **Glucose Intolerance**: People with prediabetes or undiagnosed insulin resistance may have difficulty processing glucose, leading to an increase in fat deposition in the liver and an elevated risk of developing fatty liver disease.

d) High Cholesterol and High Blood Pressure

- **Elevated Cholesterol Levels**: High levels of low-density lipoprotein (LDL) cholesterol ("bad cholesterol") contribute to the buildup of fat in the liver. The liver's role in processing fats can be hindered by elevated cholesterol levels, leading to a cycle of fat accumulation and inflammation.
- **Hypertension (High Blood Pressure)**: Chronic high blood pressure is another risk factor for fatty liver disease. It can increase the likelihood of liver inflammation and fibrosis, which may accelerate the progression of NAFLD to NASH.

e) Genetics and Family History

- **Genetic Predisposition**: Genetics play a role in the development of fatty liver disease. Certain genetic variations can make individuals more prone to storing fat in the liver or developing insulin resistance. For example, people with certain variations in the **PNPLA3 gene** are at an increased risk for developing fatty liver disease.
- **Family History**: If you have a family history of fatty liver disease, diabetes, or obesity, your risk of developing fatty liver disease increases. Genetic factors combined with lifestyle choices can amplify the chances of developing liver-related health issues.

f) Sedentary Lifestyle and Lack of Exercise

- **Physical Inactivity**: A lack of physical activity is one of the primary contributors to obesity and insulin

resistance, both of which increase the risk of fatty liver disease. Regular exercise helps reduce liver fat, improve insulin sensitivity, and promote overall metabolic health.
- **Muscle Mass and Fat Burning**: Building muscle mass through strength training exercises can improve fat metabolism. When you have more muscle, your body burns more calories and fat even while at rest, reducing the risk of fat accumulation in the liver.

g) Age and Gender

- **Age**: The risk of developing fatty liver disease increases with age, particularly after 40. Over time, liver function can decline, and the liver's ability to break down and process fat becomes less efficient.
- **Gender**: Men are at a slightly higher risk of developing fatty liver disease compared to women. However, women tend to develop more severe liver damage as they enter menopause due to hormonal changes, making post-menopausal women more susceptible.

h) Alcohol Consumption

- **Moderate to Heavy Drinking**: While NAFLD is not caused by alcohol, excessive alcohol consumption can accelerate the progression of fatty liver disease to more severe forms like NASH. Alcohol causes inflammation and oxidative stress in liver cells, which can worsen liver damage.
- **Alcohol and NAFLD**: It's important to distinguish between alcohol-related fatty liver disease (ALD) and NAFLD. ALD is caused primarily by alcohol, while

NAFLD is typically associated with non-alcoholic factors such as obesity and diabetes. However, alcohol can exacerbate existing NAFLD.

2. Common Misconceptions About Fatty Liver Disease

Despite its prevalence, there are many misconceptions about fatty liver disease that can delay diagnosis and treatment. These misunderstandings often prevent people from taking the necessary steps to protect their liver health. Let's debunk some of the most common myths:

a) "Fatty Liver Disease Only Affects Overweight People"

This is one of the most widespread misconceptions, but fatty liver disease can affect people of all body types, including those who are at a normal weight. While being overweight or obese is a major risk factor, people with normal or even low body weight can still develop fatty liver disease due to factors like insulin resistance, genetics, and poor dietary habits. In fact, lean individuals with fatty liver disease may be more likely to develop advanced liver damage, such as NASH, because they may have other underlying health issues like metabolic syndrome.

b) "You Can't Have Fatty Liver Disease If You Don't Drink Alcohol"

While it's true that excessive alcohol consumption can cause fatty liver disease (ALD), **Non-Alcoholic Fatty Liver Disease (NAFLD)** can occur without alcohol consumption. NAFLD is typically associated with metabolic risk factors such as obesity, diabetes, and high cholesterol. So, it is crucial not to assume that drinking habits are the sole cause of fatty liver disease.

c) "Fatty Liver Disease Doesn't Need to Be Treated"

Many people believe that fatty liver disease is harmless in its early stages and doesn't require medical attention. In reality, if left untreated, fatty liver disease can progress to more severe conditions like NASH, cirrhosis, and liver cancer. Early intervention through dietary changes, weight loss, and exercise can help prevent the disease from progressing and restore liver function.

d) "Only Older Adults Get Fatty Liver Disease"

Fatty liver disease is often associated with aging, but it can affect individuals of all ages, including children and teenagers. The increasing rates of childhood obesity and poor dietary habits have led to a rise in fatty liver disease among younger populations. Early intervention is key to managing fatty liver disease in both children and adults.

e) "Fatty Liver Disease Symptoms Are Always Obvious"

In many cases, fatty liver disease has no noticeable symptoms, especially in the early stages. People with the condition may not experience any pain or discomfort, which is why fatty liver disease is often referred to as a "silent disease." This is why routine screenings and blood tests are crucial for early detection, particularly for those at risk.

f) "A Fatty Liver Can Heal Itself with Time"

While it is possible to reverse early-stage fatty liver disease with lifestyle changes such as diet and exercise, the liver does not always heal on its own, especially once it progresses to more severe forms like NASH or cirrhosis. Delaying treatment or making only minimal changes can lead to irreversible liver damage, so proactive intervention is vital.

Debunking Myths About Fatty Liver Disease

Fatty liver disease (FLD), including Non-Alcoholic Fatty Liver Disease (NAFLD) and its more severe form, Non-Alcoholic Steatohepatitis (NASH), is often misunderstood due to a range of misconceptions that circulate in the public domain. These myths can prevent individuals from recognizing the importance of early intervention, understanding their risk factors, and taking proactive steps to protect their liver health. In this section, we will explore some of the most common myths about fatty liver disease and set the record straight with facts.

Myth 1: "Fatty Liver Disease Is Caused Only by Alcohol Consumption"

The Fact: While alcohol is a well-known cause of liver damage (leading to alcohol-related fatty liver disease or ALD), fatty liver disease can occur without any alcohol consumption. In fact, **Non-Alcoholic Fatty Liver Disease (NAFLD)** is the most common form of fatty liver disease, affecting millions of people worldwide, especially in those with risk factors like obesity, diabetes, and metabolic syndrome.

NAFLD develops when fat accumulates in the liver cells in the absence of significant alcohol consumption. Although the exact causes of NAFLD are still being researched, several factors contribute to its development, such as:

- **Obesity**: Excess body fat, especially visceral fat (fat around the abdominal area), is a major risk factor for NAFLD.
- **Insulin Resistance**: This is the condition where the body's cells become less responsive to insulin, often leading to higher levels of circulating glucose and fat in the liver.
- **Poor Diet**: Diets rich in sugar, refined carbohydrates, and unhealthy fats contribute to fat buildup in the liver.
- **Metabolic Syndrome**: This cluster of conditions, which includes high blood pressure, high blood sugar, and high cholesterol, increases the risk of developing fatty liver.

Thus, alcohol is not the sole cause of fatty liver disease, and it's important to recognize the role of these other lifestyle and genetic factors.

Myth 2: "Fatty Liver Disease Only Affects People Who Are Overweight"

The Fact: Although **obesity** is one of the leading risk factors for fatty liver disease, it's a misconception that only overweight individuals can develop the condition. People with a **normal body weight** can also develop **NAFLD**, especially those who have **lean fatty liver disease**. This condition occurs when fat accumulates in the liver of individuals who are not obese but still have factors like poor diet, insulin resistance, or genetic predispositions that contribute to fat buildup in the liver cells.

For example:

- **Non-obese individuals with insulin resistance**: Even lean individuals who have issues with glucose metabolism (such as those with prediabetes or metabolic syndrome) may develop fatty liver disease.
- **Genetic factors**: Certain genetic variants can increase the likelihood of fat accumulation in the liver, even in those who are not overweight. For instance, variations in the **PNPLA3 gene** are known to increase the risk of fatty liver in both obese and lean individuals.

The takeaway is that fatty liver disease can affect individuals of all sizes, so weight should not be the only factor used to assess risk.

Myth 3: "You'll Experience Symptoms Right Away"

The Fact: Fatty liver disease is often referred to as a **"silent disease"** because many people with the condition don't experience noticeable symptoms, especially in the early stages. In fact, most people with **NAFLD** do not feel pain or discomfort until the condition has progressed to more severe stages, such as **NASH** (Non-Alcoholic Steatohepatitis) or cirrhosis.

Symptoms, if they occur, may include:

- **Fatigue** or feeling tired for no clear reason
- **Abdominal discomfort** or bloating, especially in the upper right abdomen

- **Unexplained weight loss** (in later stages of the disease)
- **Dark urine** and **yellowing of the skin or eyes** (signs of advanced liver damage)

Because fatty liver disease can develop without clear symptoms, it's crucial for individuals at risk—especially those with obesity, diabetes, or a family history of liver disease—to have regular check-ups and liver function tests. Routine blood tests and imaging (like ultrasound or MRI) can help detect early signs of fatty liver disease before it becomes symptomatic or more serious.

Myth 4: "Fatty Liver Disease Isn't Dangerous Until It's Advanced"

The Fact: It's a dangerous misconception that fatty liver disease isn't serious until it's advanced. In reality, even in its early stages, fatty liver disease can be harmful. **NAFLD** may seem mild at first, but if left untreated, it can progress to more severe liver conditions, including **NASH**, **cirrhosis**, or even **liver cancer**.

- **Non-Alcoholic Steatohepatitis (NASH)** is an advanced form of NAFLD that involves inflammation and liver cell damage, which can lead to scarring (fibrosis). If NASH progresses, it can result in cirrhosis, where the liver becomes severely scarred and loses its ability to function.
- **Cirrhosis**: In the later stages of cirrhosis, the liver can become so damaged that it can no longer perform essential functions, leading to liver failure and the need for a liver transplant.

- **Liver Cancer**: Fatty liver disease, particularly in its NASH form, is also a significant risk factor for the development of liver cancer.

This is why early intervention is critical. Adopting a healthier lifestyle and managing risk factors such as obesity, diabetes, and high cholesterol can prevent the progression of the disease, even in its early stages.

Myth 5: "There's No Treatment for Fatty Liver Disease"

The Fact: While there is no single FDA-approved medication specifically for fatty liver disease, **lifestyle changes** are the cornerstone of managing and even reversing the condition. The liver has an incredible capacity for regeneration, and with the right approach, individuals can reduce liver fat, reverse inflammation, and prevent further damage.

The main treatment strategies for fatty liver disease include:

- **Dietary Changes**: A healthy, balanced diet rich in whole foods, fiber, lean proteins, healthy fats, and low in processed sugars and trans fats can significantly reduce liver fat. Focus on anti-inflammatory foods like fruits, vegetables, and foods high in antioxidants.
- **Exercise**: Regular physical activity, especially aerobic exercise, helps reduce liver fat and improve insulin sensitivity, reducing the burden on the liver.
- **Weight Loss**: Losing even a small percentage of body weight (about 5-10%) can significantly reduce liver fat and improve liver function.
- **Medications for Underlying Conditions**: Managing conditions like diabetes, high cholesterol, and high

blood pressure with the help of prescribed medications can also improve liver health.
- **Monitoring Liver Health**: Regular check-ups, blood tests, and imaging can help track liver function and monitor progress in reducing fat accumulation.

Even without specific medications, the lifestyle changes mentioned above can help people living with fatty liver disease improve their liver health and prevent progression to more severe stages.

Myth 6: "You Don't Need to Worry About Fatty Liver Disease If You Don't Have Any Symptoms"

The Fact: As mentioned earlier, fatty liver disease is often asymptomatic in its early stages. The absence of symptoms does not mean the condition isn't progressing or isn't harmful. By the time symptoms appear, the liver may have already sustained significant damage, making it harder to reverse the condition.

That's why **early detection** is essential. If you're at risk—whether due to obesity, diabetes, high blood pressure, or a family history of liver disease—it's important to undergo regular screening, even if you feel healthy. Early intervention through lifestyle changes can make a significant difference in preventing the disease from advancing.

Identifying Risk Factors for Fatty Liver Disease: Genetics, Diet, Lifestyle, and Environmental Factors

Fatty liver disease (FLD), including its most common form, **Non-Alcoholic Fatty Liver Disease (NAFLD)**, has become an increasingly prevalent health concern worldwide. Understanding the **risk factors** that contribute to the development of fatty liver is crucial for prevention and management. While certain factors are within our control—such as diet and lifestyle—others, like genetics and environmental influences, are not. A thorough understanding of these risk factors can empower individuals to take action, modify their habits, and minimize their risk of developing fatty liver disease or its more severe form, **Non-Alcoholic Steatohepatitis (NASH)**.

In this section, we will explore the key risk factors for fatty liver disease, focusing on **genetics, diet, lifestyle**, and **environmental influences**. Understanding these factors is essential for anyone who wants to take proactive steps in managing their liver health and living a healthier life.

1. Genetics: The Role of Your DNA

Genetics play a significant role in determining an individual's susceptibility to fatty liver disease. While lifestyle and environmental factors are crucial, your genetic makeup can influence how your liver handles fat metabolism, inflammation, and overall liver health. Studies have identified specific genetic factors that increase the risk of developing fatty liver disease, even in the absence of other typical risk factors like obesity or alcohol consumption.

Key Genetic Risk Factors:

- **PNPLA3 Gene**: One of the most studied genetic factors associated with NAFLD is the **PNPLA3 gene**. Certain variations of this gene are linked to an increased risk of fat accumulation in the liver. These variations are found more frequently in individuals with a higher likelihood of developing **NASH** and liver fibrosis.
- **TM6SF2 Gene**: Another important gene is **TM6SF2**, which has been shown to increase liver fat accumulation and is linked to a higher risk of severe liver damage in individuals with NAFLD.
- **MBOAT7 Gene**: This gene has been implicated in the development of liver disease, particularly in individuals who carry a specific variant. It is believed to influence the liver's ability to metabolize lipids and play a role in inflammation and fat accumulation.

Genetics also plays a role in other metabolic conditions like **obesity** and **insulin resistance**, which are themselves major risk factors for fatty liver disease. If you have a family history of fatty liver disease, **diabetes**, or other metabolic disorders, your risk of developing NAFLD or NASH may be higher.

2. Diet: The Impact of What You Eat

Diet is one of the most modifiable risk factors when it comes to preventing or managing fatty liver disease. **Poor dietary habits**—such as consuming foods high in **sugars**, **refined carbohydrates**, **saturated fats**, and **processed foods**—are strongly linked to the development of fatty liver.

Key Dietary Factors That Contribute to Fatty Liver Disease:

- **Excessive Sugar and Refined Carbohydrates**: Diets high in **added sugars** (especially fructose) and refined carbohydrates (such as white bread, pasta, and sugary beverages) are a significant contributor to the development of fatty liver disease. These foods can lead to **insulin resistance**, which is one of the primary drivers of fat buildup in the liver.
- **Saturated and Trans Fats**: A diet high in unhealthy fats—especially **saturated fats** (found in fatty cuts of meat, butter, and full-fat dairy) and **trans fats** (found in processed snacks, fast food, and margarine)—can exacerbate fat accumulation in the liver. These fats promote inflammation and oxidative stress, both of which contribute to liver damage and fibrosis.
- **Lack of Fiber**: Diets low in fiber, which is commonly found in fruits, vegetables, and whole grains, can lead to poor liver health. **Fiber** helps regulate blood sugar levels and reduce the amount of fat deposited in the liver.
- **Alcohol**: While alcohol consumption is not the primary cause of **NAFLD**, excessive drinking can lead to alcoholic fatty liver disease (AFLD), which can coexist with non-alcoholic fatty liver. It's important to understand the difference, especially if someone has an unhealthy relationship with alcohol.

Healthy Dietary Habits to Reduce Risk:

- **Increase Antioxidant-Rich Foods**: Fruits and vegetables are rich in **antioxidants** that can reduce liver inflammation and oxidative stress. Berries, leafy

greens, cruciferous vegetables (like broccoli and cauliflower), and citrus fruits are excellent choices.
- **Eat Healthy Fats**: Incorporating **omega-3 fatty acids** from sources like **fatty fish** (salmon, sardines), flaxseeds, and walnuts can help reduce liver fat accumulation and inflammation.
- **Whole Grains**: Opt for **whole grains** like quinoa, brown rice, oats, and barley, which provide fiber that helps improve liver function and insulin sensitivity.
- **Moderate Protein**: Choose lean sources of protein, such as chicken, fish, legumes, and plant-based proteins, over processed meats that are high in unhealthy fats.

3. Lifestyle: Physical Activity and Weight Management

Your lifestyle choices, particularly **physical activity** and **weight management**, play an integral role in preventing and managing fatty liver disease. Research shows that **regular exercise** can improve liver function, reduce fat accumulation, and combat inflammation in the liver. In fact, a combination of **a healthy diet** and **exercise** is often the most effective approach for reversing or managing fatty liver disease.

Key Lifestyle Factors That Affect Liver Health:

- **Obesity**: Obesity, particularly excess fat around the abdomen (visceral fat), is one of the most significant risk factors for fatty liver disease. The accumulation of fat in the liver is directly linked to insulin resistance and metabolic dysfunction, which in turn contributes to liver damage.

- **Physical Inactivity**: A sedentary lifestyle—characterized by sitting for long periods and lack of physical activity—can increase the likelihood of fat buildup in the liver. Regular exercise helps improve insulin sensitivity, promote weight loss, and reduce liver fat.
- **Stress**: Chronic stress can lead to unhealthy lifestyle choices, such as overeating, poor food choices, and inactivity, all of which can exacerbate fatty liver disease. Stress also triggers the release of hormones like **cortisol**, which can increase fat storage in the liver.
- **Sleep**: **Sleep disorders**, such as sleep apnea, are linked to an increased risk of developing fatty liver disease. Poor sleep can disrupt metabolic processes and promote weight gain, particularly abdominal fat.

Lifestyle Changes to Reduce Risk:

- **Regular Exercise**: Aim for **at least 150 minutes of moderate-intensity aerobic exercise** (such as brisk walking, swimming, or cycling) per week, combined with **strength training** exercises. Exercise helps reduce liver fat and improves overall metabolic health.
- **Weight Loss**: Losing **5-10% of your body weight** can significantly reduce fat in the liver, improve insulin sensitivity, and reduce inflammation. Weight loss also helps lower blood sugar and cholesterol levels.
- **Stress Management**: Practices like **meditation**, **yoga**, and **deep breathing exercises** can help manage stress, improve sleep, and promote overall well-being.

4. Environmental Factors: Toxins and Chemicals

Environmental factors can also contribute to the development of fatty liver disease. Exposure to **toxins**, **chemicals**, and other pollutants in the air, water, and food supply may have detrimental effects on liver health. Additionally, certain medications and health conditions that affect the liver can increase the risk of developing fatty liver disease.

Key Environmental Factors That Affect Liver Health:

- **Toxins and Pollutants**: Long-term exposure to environmental pollutants, such as heavy metals, industrial chemicals, and pesticides, has been shown to increase the risk of liver disease. These substances can cause oxidative stress and inflammation, contributing to liver damage.
- **Medications**: Certain medications, including corticosteroids, antiretroviral drugs, and some cancer treatments, can lead to **drug-induced liver injury**, which increases the risk of fatty liver disease.
- **Hormonal Imbalances**: Environmental factors that disrupt hormonal balance, such as **endocrine-disrupting chemicals** (found in plastics and personal care products), may contribute to the development of fatty liver disease by promoting fat accumulation and liver inflammation.

Why Diet Matters for Liver Health

The liver is one of the most vital organs in the body, responsible for detoxification, metabolism, digestion, and nutrient storage. It plays a central role in processing the food and beverages we consume, filtering toxins, and regulating blood sugar levels. What we eat has a profound effect on how well the liver functions. **Dietary choices** can either support liver health or contribute to conditions like **fatty liver disease** (NAFLD), **non-alcoholic steatohepatitis** (NASH), and other liver disorders. Therefore, understanding the relationship between diet and liver health is crucial for both the prevention and management of liver diseases.

In this chapter, we will explore why **diet matters** for liver health, how certain foods can protect or damage the liver, and how making the right dietary choices can lead to a healthier liver and a healthier life.

1. The Liver's Role in Metabolism

The liver is essential in regulating the body's metabolism, which includes converting food into usable energy, storing nutrients, and synthesizing proteins. When the liver's capacity to perform these functions is compromised, such as in the case of **fatty liver disease**, the body's metabolic processes become unbalanced, leading to inflammation, fat accumulation, and even fibrosis (scarring). A poor diet that includes excessive amounts of sugar, unhealthy fats, and processed foods can impair the liver's ability to do its job effectively.

How Diet Affects Metabolism:

- **Sugar and Carbohydrates**: Consuming an excessive amount of **added sugars** (especially fructose) and refined carbohydrates (white bread, pasta, and sugary

beverages) leads to an increase in **insulin resistance**. When the liver is overwhelmed by too much sugar, it stores the excess as fat, contributing to **fatty liver** and increasing the risk of developing metabolic syndrome and Type 2 diabetes.
- **Unhealthy Fats**: Diets rich in **saturated fats** and **trans fats** (found in fast food, processed snacks, and margarine) disrupt the liver's ability to metabolize fats properly. These fats are harder for the liver to process, and over time, they can accumulate in liver cells, leading to **non-alcoholic fatty liver disease (NAFLD)**.
- **Insulin Resistance**: A diet high in sugar and processed foods can lead to **insulin resistance**, a key factor in fatty liver disease. When insulin resistance occurs, the liver becomes less responsive to insulin, causing it to accumulate excess fat and impairing its ability to regulate blood sugar.

2. The Impact of Fatty Foods on Liver Function

While the liver plays a critical role in processing dietary fats, excessive intake of certain types of fat can overwhelm its capacity. In particular, **saturated fats**, found in red meat, butter, and full-fat dairy, and **trans fats**, commonly found in packaged baked goods, fried foods, and fast foods, can have damaging effects on liver health.

Effects of Unhealthy Fats on the Liver:

- **Fat Accumulation**: When the liver is overloaded with fats, it begins to store them inside liver cells, leading to **fatty liver disease**. This excess fat disrupts the normal

functioning of liver cells, triggering inflammation, which can progress to **non-alcoholic steatohepatitis (NASH)**, a more serious form of liver damage.
- **Increased Inflammation**: Saturated and trans fats promote the production of **inflammatory molecules** that damage liver cells and contribute to the progression of fatty liver disease. Chronic inflammation can also lead to fibrosis (scarring) of the liver tissue, which can eventually progress to cirrhosis and liver failure if not addressed.
- **Oxidative Stress**: High-fat diets can increase **oxidative stress** in the liver, which damages liver cells and accelerates the development of liver diseases. This oxidative damage occurs when there is an imbalance between free radicals (harmful molecules) and antioxidants in the liver, and it plays a significant role in the progression of fatty liver disease.

3. The Role of Fiber and Whole Foods in Liver Health

A diet high in **fiber** and **whole foods** is essential for maintaining optimal liver function. Fiber, found in fruits, vegetables, whole grains, and legumes, helps the body digest food more effectively, regulate blood sugar, and support overall digestive health. It also promotes liver detoxification, aiding the liver in clearing out waste products and toxins from the body.

How Fiber Protects the Liver:

- **Improved Insulin Sensitivity**: Fiber helps improve insulin sensitivity by slowing down the absorption of

sugars into the bloodstream. This helps regulate blood sugar levels, reducing the burden on the liver and minimizing the risk of fatty liver disease.
- **Detoxification**: Fiber promotes the elimination of waste products from the body. It binds to toxins in the digestive system, helping to prevent their reabsorption and assisting the liver in its detoxification process.
- **Weight Management**: A high-fiber diet can help with weight management by promoting feelings of fullness and reducing overall calorie intake. Maintaining a healthy weight is crucial for reducing the risk of fatty liver disease, as excess body fat, particularly visceral fat, is closely linked to liver fat accumulation.
- **Reduction of Inflammation**: Fiber-rich foods are also high in antioxidants, which reduce liver inflammation. Antioxidants like vitamins C and E, found in fruits and vegetables, combat the oxidative stress caused by a poor diet and protect the liver from damage.

4. Nutrients That Support Liver Health

In addition to fiber, certain nutrients play a crucial role in supporting liver health and preventing fatty liver disease. A well-balanced diet rich in vitamins, minerals, and healthy fats provides the liver with the tools it needs to function properly.

Essential Nutrients for Liver Health:

- **Omega-3 Fatty Acids**: Found in fatty fish like salmon, sardines, and mackerel, omega-3 fatty acids have anti-inflammatory properties that help reduce liver fat accumulation. Omega-3s also improve insulin

sensitivity and reduce triglyceride levels, both of which are beneficial for liver health.
- **Vitamin E**: This powerful antioxidant has been shown to reduce liver inflammation and oxidative stress. Studies suggest that vitamin E may help reduce the severity of fatty liver disease, particularly in people with NASH. Good sources of vitamin E include nuts, seeds, and green leafy vegetables.
- **Vitamin D**: There is growing evidence that vitamin D deficiency is associated with an increased risk of fatty liver disease and its progression. Ensuring adequate levels of vitamin D—through sun exposure, fortified foods, and supplements—may help prevent and manage fatty liver.
- **B Vitamins**: B vitamins, particularly B12, folate, and B6, play a vital role in liver detoxification and fat metabolism. A deficiency in these vitamins can impair liver function and contribute to fatty liver disease. Foods rich in B vitamins include eggs, legumes, leafy greens, and whole grains.

5. Hydration: The Often Overlooked Factor

While food is critical for liver health, proper hydration is also an essential but often overlooked component. The liver needs water to carry out its functions, including detoxification and the breakdown of fats. Dehydration can impair liver function, making it harder for the body to process and eliminate toxins, and can contribute to liver stress.

The Importance of Staying Hydrated:

- **Toxin Elimination**: Water helps the liver flush out waste products and toxins from the body, preventing a buildup that could lead to liver damage.
- **Metabolism Support**: Staying hydrated supports the liver's role in metabolizing fats and sugars, reducing the risk of fat accumulation in the liver.
- **Reducing Inflammation**: Proper hydration also helps reduce liver inflammation by maintaining optimal liver function and supporting overall cellular health.

6. Diet Tips for Maintaining a Healthy Liver

- **Limit Sugary and Processed Foods**: Avoid excessive amounts of added sugars, refined carbohydrates, and processed foods. Focus on whole, natural foods that nourish the liver and body.
- **Eat Healthy Fats**: Incorporate more **monounsaturated fats** and **omega-3 fatty acids** into your diet. Sources include olive oil, avocados, nuts, seeds, and fatty fish.
- **Prioritize Fiber-Rich Foods**: Include more fruits, vegetables, whole grains, and legumes in your meals. These foods provide fiber, antioxidants, and essential nutrients that support liver health.
- **Stay Hydrated**: Drink plenty of water throughout the day. Aim for at least 8 cups of water a day, and more if you are physically active.
- **Moderation**: While certain foods can support liver health, moderation is key. Avoid overeating and try to

maintain a balanced diet that includes a variety of nutrient-dense foods.

How the Food We Eat Directly Impacts Liver Function

The liver is a powerhouse organ that plays a crucial role in over 500 vital functions in the body, from detoxification and metabolism to nutrient storage and digestion. It acts as a filter for toxins, processes fats and carbohydrates, regulates blood sugar, synthesizes proteins, and stores vitamins and minerals. Given its critical role, maintaining liver health is paramount for overall well-being.

One of the most important factors influencing liver health is **diet**. The foods we consume can either support the liver's functions or place additional strain on it, contributing to the development of **fatty liver disease** (NAFLD), **cirrhosis**, and other liver conditions. In this chapter, we will explore how the food we eat directly impacts liver function, both positively and negatively, and why making conscious dietary choices can be a game-changer for liver health.

1. The Liver's Role in Processing Food and Nutrients

Before diving into the specifics of how food affects liver health, it's important to understand the liver's role in digesting and processing the food we eat. Every time you eat, your liver is hard at work breaking down the nutrients in the food, processing fats and carbohydrates, converting toxins into less harmful substances, and helping the body maintain a stable balance of essential nutrients.

The Liver's Primary Functions in Digestion and Metabolism:

- **Carbohydrate Metabolism**: The liver helps regulate blood sugar by converting excess glucose into glycogen for storage. It also releases glucose into the bloodstream when needed to keep blood sugar levels stable.
- **Fat Metabolism**: After fats are broken down in the digestive system, the liver metabolizes them, producing essential fatty acids and cholesterol that are used throughout the body. The liver also stores fat-soluble vitamins like A, D, E, and K.
- **Protein Synthesis**: The liver synthesizes proteins necessary for blood clotting, immune function, and cell repair, and it also processes amino acids from dietary proteins.
- **Detoxification**: The liver detoxifies harmful substances that enter the body, such as alcohol, medications, and environmental toxins. It processes these toxins into water-soluble compounds that can be safely excreted through the urine or bile.

As you can see, the liver is constantly at work to keep your body balanced. The food you eat can either aid in this process or overwhelm the liver's capacity to function effectively.

2. The Impact of Diet on Liver Function

Certain foods and nutrients can either promote liver health or damage it. The relationship between diet and liver function is intricate, with both **nutrients** and **toxins** affecting the liver in profound ways. Let's explore how specific dietary choices can directly impact the liver:

Dietary Impact on Fatty Liver Disease:

- **Excess Sugar and Refined Carbohydrates**: Diets high in **added sugars** and **refined carbs** (found in white bread, pasta, sugary beverages, and processed snacks) are directly linked to the development of **non-alcoholic fatty liver disease** (NAFLD). When consumed in excess, sugar (particularly fructose) and refined carbs can cause the liver to store fat, leading to fatty liver. This condition is associated with insulin resistance, high triglycerides, and an increased risk of Type 2 diabetes. The liver's ability to process fats is compromised, and fat accumulates in liver cells.
- **Unhealthy Fats**: Saturated fats (found in fatty cuts of meat, butter, and full-fat dairy) and **trans fats** (found in fried foods and many processed snacks) can have a direct, negative effect on liver health. These fats are more difficult for the liver to break down, causing fat to accumulate in the liver cells, resulting in **fatty liver disease** and increasing the risk of inflammation, fibrosis, and cirrhosis.

Positive Impact of Healthy Fats:

In contrast, **healthy fats** like **omega-3 fatty acids** (found in fatty fish like salmon, sardines, and mackerel) and **monounsaturated fats** (found in olive oil, avocado, and nuts) help reduce inflammation, improve insulin sensitivity, and promote fat breakdown in the liver. Omega-3s, in particular, have been shown to reduce liver fat content and improve overall liver function.

3. Toxins in Food and Their Effect on the Liver

Every time you eat, your liver works to process the food, but it also has to deal with the toxins present in food. Over time, consuming foods with harmful additives, pesticides, or excessive alcohol can damage liver cells and increase the risk of liver diseases. Here's how some common food toxins can affect liver health:

- **Alcohol**: One of the most well-known substances that impact liver function is **alcohol**. Excessive alcohol consumption leads to **alcoholic fatty liver disease (AFLD)**, which can progress to alcoholic hepatitis and cirrhosis. Alcohol is metabolized in the liver, and excessive consumption causes the liver to become inflamed and unable to process fats, resulting in fat accumulation and liver damage.
- **Pesticides and Chemicals**: Non-organic produce may contain pesticide residues, which the liver must process and detoxify. Chronic exposure to these chemicals can overwhelm the liver, causing **liver toxicity** and impairing liver function. **Food additives** like artificial sweeteners, preservatives, and colorants can also burden the liver over time.
- **Heavy Metals**: Certain foods, particularly fish, can contain harmful levels of heavy metals like mercury, which accumulate in the liver and can contribute to liver toxicity and damage.

4. How Nutrients Support or Impair Liver Function

While some foods can have a negative impact on liver function, other foods and nutrients are essential for supporting liver health. Here are some key nutrients and how they help the liver:

Beneficial Nutrients for Liver Health:

- **Fiber**: A diet rich in **fiber** from fruits, vegetables, whole grains, and legumes helps support liver health by promoting digestion, stabilizing blood sugar levels, and aiding in detoxification. Fiber also helps reduce liver inflammation and fat accumulation by improving insulin sensitivity.
- **Antioxidants**: Foods high in **antioxidants**—such as vitamins A, C, and E—protect liver cells from oxidative damage caused by free radicals. Antioxidants help reduce inflammation in the liver and protect it from further damage. Fruits, vegetables, nuts, seeds, and leafy greens are excellent sources of antioxidants.
- **B Vitamins**: B vitamins, particularly **B12**, **B6**, and **folate**, play a vital role in liver detoxification and fat metabolism. Deficiencies in B vitamins can hinder the liver's ability to process fats and detoxify the body effectively.
- **Vitamin D**: Emerging research suggests that **vitamin D** deficiency may be linked to an increased risk of fatty liver disease. Vitamin D helps reduce liver inflammation and improve insulin sensitivity, making it essential for liver health. Sources of vitamin D include sunlight, fortified foods, and fatty fish.

The Importance of Protein for Liver Repair:

- **Amino Acids**: The liver also requires **amino acids** (the building blocks of protein) to repair damaged liver cells. A diet that provides adequate protein from sources like lean meats, legumes, nuts, and seeds helps maintain liver health and promotes tissue regeneration.

5. Why A Balanced Diet is Essential for Liver Health

A **balanced diet** is essential for maintaining optimal liver function and preventing liver disease. When we eat, we should focus on consuming a variety of nutrient-dense foods that support liver detoxification, reduce inflammation, and maintain a healthy weight. Eating whole, unprocessed foods while limiting unhealthy fats, added sugars, and refined carbohydrates helps prevent fat buildup in the liver and promotes efficient liver function.

Some **dietary guidelines** for supporting liver health include:

- **Prioritize whole foods**: Focus on **whole grains**, **fruits**, **vegetables**, and **lean proteins** that provide essential vitamins, minerals, and fiber.
- **Healthy fats**: Include sources of **omega-3 fatty acids** and **monounsaturated fats** to reduce inflammation and support liver function.
- **Limit processed foods and sugars**: Avoid highly processed foods, sugary drinks, and refined carbohydrates that can contribute to fat buildup in the liver and insulin resistance.

- **Stay hydrated**: Drinking plenty of water is essential for detoxification and supporting liver health.
- **Avoid excessive alcohol**: Alcohol can overwhelm the liver, leading to **fatty liver** and more serious liver conditions like cirrhosis and liver failure.

Chapter 2: The Science of Reversing Fatty Liver – What Works and What Doesn't

Fatty liver disease, particularly **non-alcoholic fatty liver disease** (NAFLD), is one of the most common liver disorders worldwide. The good news is that in its early stages, fatty liver is **reversible**. The key to reversing the condition lies in understanding the science behind it and knowing which strategies are proven to work and which ones don't. In this chapter, we will explore the scientific mechanisms of fatty liver disease, how lifestyle and diet play pivotal roles in its reversal, and provide evidence-based approaches to restoring liver health.

1. Understanding the Mechanism of Fatty Liver Disease

Before diving into the methods of reversing fatty liver, it's important to first understand **how fatty liver develops**. The liver, like all organs, functions optimally when in a state of balance. However, factors like poor diet, sedentary lifestyle, and genetics can disrupt this balance, leading to the accumulation of excess fat in liver cells.

What Happens in Fatty Liver Disease:

- **Fat Accumulation**: The liver is responsible for metabolizing and storing nutrients, including fats. However, when the body takes in more **calories** (especially from fats, sugars, and refined carbohydrates) than it can burn, these extra calories are

stored as fat in the liver. This fat buildup leads to **steatosis**, the medical term for fatty liver.
- **Insulin Resistance**: One of the main drivers of fatty liver disease is **insulin resistance**. When the liver becomes resistant to insulin, it struggles to process glucose and fats properly. As a result, fat starts to accumulate in liver cells, which contributes to the development of fatty liver. Over time, this can lead to liver inflammation, liver damage, and the progression to more serious conditions like **non-alcoholic steatohepatitis (NASH)** and cirrhosis.
- **Inflammation and Liver Damage**: As fat accumulates in liver cells, it can cause **inflammation**. This inflammation damages liver cells, which triggers the body's immune response and further accelerates liver injury. In the advanced stages of fatty liver disease, fibrosis (scarring of liver tissue) may develop, leading to irreversible liver damage.

2. The Role of Diet in Reversing Fatty Liver

One of the most effective and scientifically supported ways to reverse fatty liver disease is through **dietary changes**. The liver's ability to process fat and glucose depends largely on the types of food we consume. Certain foods can help reduce liver fat, lower inflammation, and improve overall liver function. Here's how different dietary strategies can help:

What Works:

- **Low-Carb, High-Fiber Diet**: Studies have shown that a **low-carbohydrate, high-fiber diet** can significantly reduce liver fat content. Reducing refined sugars and starches (such as white bread, pastries, and sugary drinks) lowers the body's insulin response, which in turn reduces fat storage in the liver. Replacing refined carbs with **whole grains**, **vegetables**, **legumes**, and **fruits** provides fiber, which helps improve insulin sensitivity and liver function.

- **Anti-Inflammatory Foods**: **Inflammation** is one of the hallmarks of fatty liver disease. To counteract this, incorporating **anti-inflammatory foods** like **omega-3 fatty acids** (from fatty fish like salmon, mackerel, and sardines), **nuts**, and **seeds** can help lower liver inflammation. Omega-3s are particularly effective at reducing liver fat content and improving insulin sensitivity, making them essential for liver recovery.
- **Weight Loss**: The most proven method to reverse fatty liver disease is **weight loss**. Research has shown that even a **5-10% reduction in body weight** can significantly reduce liver fat and inflammation. This is because losing weight helps improve insulin sensitivity, decreases fat storage in the liver, and reduces overall inflammation. While this can be achieved through both diet and exercise, the focus should be on losing weight gradually (1-2 pounds per week) for long-term liver health benefits.
- **Antioxidant-Rich Foods**: The liver is constantly working to detoxify harmful substances in the body. **Antioxidants** help protect liver cells from oxidative damage caused by toxins and free radicals. Foods rich in antioxidants, such as **berries**, **leafy greens**, **green tea**, and **cruciferous vegetables** (e.g., broccoli, Brussels sprouts, and kale), help reduce oxidative stress, lower liver inflammation, and promote liver regeneration.

What Doesn't Work:

- **Crash Diets or Extreme Caloric Restriction**: While weight loss is essential for reversing fatty liver, **extreme dieting or rapid weight loss** can actually worsen liver health. Rapid weight loss may lead to a condition known as **fatty liver-related liver damage**, where the liver releases stored fats too quickly into the bloodstream, potentially worsening fat accumulation in liver cells. The key is gradual, sustainable weight loss.
- **Eliminating All Fats**: While unhealthy fats (like trans fats and excessive saturated fats) should be avoided, completely eliminating all fats from the diet is not recommended. Healthy fats, particularly **omega-3 fatty acids**, are crucial for reducing liver inflammation and improving liver function. A diet too low in fat can also disrupt the absorption of fat-soluble vitamins (A, D, E, K) that are vital for overall health.

3. The Science Behind Exercise and Fatty Liver Reversal

Exercise plays a critical role in reversing fatty liver disease. Regular physical activity improves insulin sensitivity, reduces liver fat, and promotes overall metabolic health. But how exactly does exercise work in helping the liver?

What Works:

- **Aerobic Exercise**: **Aerobic exercises**, such as walking, jogging, cycling, or swimming, have been shown to significantly reduce liver fat. Regular aerobic activity

increases the body's ability to burn fat, reduces insulin resistance, and lowers inflammation. Studies suggest that even moderate-intensity exercise for at least **30 minutes, 5 times a week** can improve liver health in individuals with fatty liver disease.
- **Strength Training**: **Strength training** or resistance exercises (such as weightlifting or bodyweight exercises) also support liver health by increasing muscle mass, improving metabolic rate, and enhancing fat burning. When combined with aerobic exercise, strength training can further improve insulin sensitivity and help with weight management, both of which are crucial for reversing fatty liver.

What Doesn't Work:

- **Excessive Exercise**: While regular physical activity is key to reversing fatty liver, **over-exercising** (especially without proper rest and recovery) can place additional strain on the body, leading to stress-induced **inflammation**. This can be counterproductive for liver health. It is important to balance exercise with adequate rest and recovery.

4. Medical Interventions for Fatty Liver Disease

While lifestyle changes such as diet and exercise are the cornerstone of reversing fatty liver disease, some people may need **medical intervention** depending on the severity of their condition. Medications may be prescribed to manage risk factors such as high cholesterol, high blood sugar, or high blood pressure. However, there is currently no specific medication approved for the treatment of fatty liver disease.

What Works:

- **Managing Underlying Conditions**: Treating **insulin resistance**, **obesity**, **diabetes**, and **high cholesterol** through medications prescribed by a healthcare provider can be beneficial in reversing fatty liver disease. For example, medications like **metformin** or **glitazones** can improve insulin sensitivity, while **statins** may help control cholesterol levels.

What Doesn't Work:

- **Unproven Supplements**: Many supplements and alternative treatments claim to "cure" or "reverse" fatty liver disease. However, there is limited evidence to support the effectiveness of many of these supplements. While some herbs and supplements (like **milk thistle** and **turmeric**) may offer some liver-protective benefits, they are not a substitute for a balanced diet, exercise, and medical care.
- **Fad Detox Programs**: Detox diets and cleanses that promise to "flush out" liver fat are generally ineffective for long-term liver health. The liver itself is already highly efficient at detoxifying the body, and while a healthy diet may support its function, extreme detox programs can disrupt the body's natural processes and worsen liver function.

5. Creating a Holistic Approach to Liver Health

The science of reversing fatty liver disease lies in a **comprehensive approach** that involves diet, exercise, lifestyle modifications, and medical management. A balanced diet rich in whole foods, healthy fats, fiber, and antioxidants, combined with regular physical activity, is essential to restore liver function and reduce fat accumulation in the liver.

Tips for a Holistic Approach:

- **Prioritize whole, unprocessed foods** and minimize added sugars, refined carbs, and unhealthy fats.
- **Incorporate regular physical activity**, combining both aerobic and strength training exercises.
- **Manage stress** through relaxation techniques like yoga or mindfulness to reduce inflammation and support liver recovery.
- **Stay hydrated** and avoid alcohol, which can damage liver cells.
- **Consult a healthcare professional** for regular liver function tests and to manage any underlying health conditions such as diabetes or hypertension.

The Healing Power of Nutrition: Scientifically-Backed Foods That Heal the Liver

The liver is one of the most resilient organs in the body, capable of regenerating itself even after significant damage. However, when the liver is under constant strain—due to factors like poor diet, alcohol consumption, environmental toxins, and chronic illnesses—its ability to heal diminishes.

The good news is that proper nutrition can play a pivotal role in healing and supporting liver function. In this section, we will discuss scientifically-backed foods and nutrients that can help heal the liver, including antioxidants, healthy fats, and specific vitamins and minerals like **Vitamin E, omega-3 fatty acids**, and **fiber**.

1. The Role of Antioxidants in Liver Health

The liver is the body's primary detoxification organ. It filters toxins, processes fats, and produces important substances like bile and proteins. However, this heavy workload creates **oxidative stress**—a condition where the body produces an excess of free radicals (unstable molecules that damage cells) and struggles to neutralize them. Oxidative stress is a significant contributor to liver inflammation, fatty liver disease, and even liver fibrosis.

How Antioxidants Help:

Antioxidants are compounds that help neutralize free radicals and reduce oxidative stress, thus protecting liver cells from damage. A diet rich in antioxidant-rich foods can support the liver's detoxification process and reduce inflammation, both of which are key to maintaining or restoring liver health.

- **Vitamin C**: This powerful antioxidant is known for its ability to reduce oxidative stress and support liver detoxification. Vitamin C-rich foods, such as citrus fruits (oranges, lemons), berries (strawberries, blueberries), and bell peppers, help regenerate other antioxidants in the body, enhancing liver protection.

- **Vitamin E**: Vitamin E is another potent antioxidant that plays a crucial role in protecting the liver from oxidative damage. It has been shown to reduce liver inflammation, particularly in those with non-alcoholic fatty liver disease (NAFLD) and non-alcoholic steatohepatitis (NASH). Foods rich in Vitamin E, such as **almonds**, **sunflower seeds**, **spinach**, and **avocados**, are key to supporting liver health.
- **Polyphenols**: These are plant-based compounds found in foods like **green tea**, **berries**, **apples**, and **dark chocolate**. Research has shown that polyphenols, particularly in green tea, have anti-inflammatory and antioxidant properties that can protect the liver from damage, enhance fat metabolism, and even help reduce fat accumulation in the liver.
- **Flavonoids**: Another group of antioxidants, flavonoids are abundant in **apples**, **onions**, **citrus fruits**, and **dark leafy greens**. Studies suggest that flavonoids help reduce oxidative stress and improve liver function, making them excellent additions to any liver-healthy diet.

2. Healthy Fats for Liver Healing

Fats are often vilified in modern diets, but not all fats are created equal. In fact, certain types of fats are essential for liver function and healing, particularly **omega-3 fatty acids**.

Omega-3 Fatty Acids:

Omega-3 fatty acids are polyunsaturated fats that are particularly beneficial for liver health. These fats have been shown to **reduce inflammation** and **lower liver fat content**. They also improve **insulin sensitivity**, which is crucial for those with fatty liver disease. Omega-3s can help decrease fat accumulation in the liver, protect liver cells from damage, and reduce overall inflammation throughout the body.

- **Sources of Omega-3s**: Fatty fish like **salmon, mackerel, sardines**, and **herring** are among the best sources of omega-3s. If you're not a fan of fish, **flaxseeds, chia seeds**, and **walnuts** also provide plant-based omega-3s, though in a slightly different form (ALA, which the body must convert to the more active forms, EPA and DHA).
- **Anti-Inflammatory Effects**: Omega-3s have been shown to reduce liver inflammation, particularly in individuals with NAFLD and NASH. Studies indicate that consuming omega-3-rich foods regularly can reduce liver fat and improve liver enzyme levels, thus helping to prevent further liver damage.

Monounsaturated Fats:

Monounsaturated fats, found in foods like **olive oil, avocados**, and **nuts**, can also benefit the liver. These healthy fats have been shown to improve lipid profiles (reduce harmful LDL cholesterol), enhance liver function, and reduce the accumulation of fat in the liver.

- **Olive Oil**: One of the best sources of monounsaturated fats, olive oil has anti-inflammatory properties that promote liver health. Extra virgin olive oil, in particular, contains **oleocanthal**, a compound that has been shown to reduce inflammation in liver cells and improve fat metabolism.

3. Fiber: The Unsung Hero for Liver Health

Fiber is one of the most important yet often overlooked nutrients for liver health. It not only supports **digestive health** but also helps the liver by reducing fat accumulation, improving insulin sensitivity, and promoting the elimination of toxins from the body.

How Fiber Supports the Liver:

- **Regulates Blood Sugar**: Fiber helps slow down the absorption of sugar into the bloodstream, preventing spikes in blood glucose levels. This is particularly important for people with **insulin resistance**, which is a major risk factor for developing fatty liver disease. By improving blood sugar regulation, fiber helps reduce fat storage in the liver and lowers the risk of developing fatty liver disease.
- **Supports Healthy Bile Production**: Bile, produced by the liver, helps digest fats and eliminates toxins from the body. **Soluble fiber** (found in foods like oats, legumes, apples, and carrots) helps bind bile acids in the digestive tract and promotes their excretion. This stimulates the liver to produce more bile, which not only aids digestion but also supports detoxification.
- **Promotes Healthy Gut Flora**: **Gut health** is deeply linked to liver health. A healthy gut microbiome plays a crucial role in regulating liver function. Fiber-rich foods help feed beneficial gut bacteria, promoting a balanced

microbiome. Research has shown that an imbalance in gut bacteria (dysbiosis) can lead to liver inflammation and fatty liver disease. By fostering a healthy gut flora, fiber indirectly supports liver function and healing.

Best Sources of Fiber for Liver Health:

- **Whole grains**: Brown rice, quinoa, barley, and oats
- **Legumes**: Lentils, chickpeas, beans, and peas
- **Fruits**: Apples, berries, pears, and citrus fruits
- **Vegetables**: Leafy greens, cruciferous vegetables (broccoli, Brussels sprouts), and root vegetables (sweet potatoes, carrots)

4. The Power of Vitamin E for Liver Health

Vitamin E is a fat-soluble antioxidant that plays a crucial role in protecting liver cells from oxidative stress and inflammation. It's particularly beneficial for individuals with **non-alcoholic steatohepatitis (NASH)**, an advanced form of fatty liver disease characterized by inflammation and liver cell damage.

How Vitamin E Helps:

- **Reduces Liver Inflammation**: Clinical studies have shown that **Vitamin E supplementation** can significantly reduce liver inflammation in people with NASH. This reduction in inflammation can help prevent the progression of fatty liver disease to more severe conditions, such as liver fibrosis or cirrhosis.
- **Protects Liver Cells**: Vitamin E works as a powerful antioxidant to protect liver cells from damage caused by

free radicals. By scavenging these harmful molecules, Vitamin E helps preserve liver cell integrity, ensuring that the liver functions optimally.

Sources of Vitamin E:

- **Nuts and seeds**: Almonds, sunflower seeds, and hazelnuts
- **Vegetable oils**: Sunflower oil, olive oil, and safflower oil
- **Leafy greens**: Spinach, Swiss chard, and kale
- **Fortified foods**: Some breakfast cereals, plant-based milks, and juices are fortified with Vitamin E

5. Putting It All Together: A Liver-Healthy Diet

To support the healing of the liver, it's essential to include a combination of the nutrients discussed above in your diet. A well-rounded approach to liver health would include:

- **A variety of antioxidant-rich foods**: Berries, citrus fruits, leafy greens, and cruciferous vegetables.
- **Healthy fats**: Omega-3s from fatty fish, flaxseeds, and walnuts; monounsaturated fats from olive oil and avocados.
- **Fiber-rich foods**: Whole grains, legumes, fruits, and vegetables.
- **Vitamin E**: From nuts, seeds, and green leafy vegetables.

Incorporating these foods into your daily diet, along with other lifestyle changes like maintaining a healthy weight, staying hydrated, and exercising regularly, will give your liver the best chance at healing and regenerating.

Understanding the Role of Insulin Resistance: The Link Between Fatty Liver and Diabetes

Insulin resistance is a critical metabolic dysfunction that has significant implications for overall health, especially when it comes to **fatty liver disease** and **diabetes**. The relationship between insulin resistance, fatty liver, and diabetes is intricate and complex, with each condition often fueling the progression of the others. In this section, we will explore how insulin resistance develops, how it impacts liver function, and its connection to the development of both non-alcoholic fatty liver disease (NAFLD) and type 2 diabetes.

1. What Is Insulin Resistance?

At its core, **insulin resistance** is a condition in which the body's cells—especially muscle, fat, and liver cells—become less responsive to the effects of insulin. Insulin is a hormone produced by the pancreas that helps cells take up glucose (sugar) from the bloodstream to use as energy or store for later. When insulin resistance occurs, the body's cells require more insulin to achieve the same effect. As a result, the pancreas produces extra insulin to compensate for the reduced efficiency.

Over time, this **increased insulin production** can lead to higher-than-normal levels of insulin in the blood, a condition called **hyperinsulinemia**. This is a key factor in the development of metabolic diseases, including fatty liver and diabetes.

2. The Link Between Insulin Resistance and Fatty Liver Disease

The liver plays a central role in regulating blood sugar levels and fat metabolism. Under normal circumstances, insulin helps the liver store excess glucose as glycogen and control the release of glucose into the bloodstream when needed. However, in the presence of insulin resistance, the liver's response to insulin is impaired, leading to several detrimental effects that directly contribute to fatty liver disease.

How Insulin Resistance Leads to Fatty Liver:

- **Increased Fat Storage in the Liver**: When insulin resistance develops, the liver's ability to effectively take up and process glucose is diminished. As a result, the liver starts converting excess glucose into fat, which is then stored in liver cells. This excess fat accumulation in the liver is the hallmark of **non-alcoholic fatty liver disease (NAFLD)**.
- **Increased Lipolysis and Fatty Acid Release**: Insulin resistance also affects the way the body processes and stores fat. In people with insulin resistance, fat cells (adipocytes) are less responsive to insulin's inhibitory effects, leading to **increased lipolysis**—the breakdown of stored fat into free fatty acids. These free fatty acids are then released into the bloodstream and delivered to the liver. This **flood of fatty acids** contributes to the

accumulation of fat in liver cells, worsening fatty liver disease.
- **Impaired Liver Fatty Acid Metabolism**: The liver is responsible for metabolizing fats, and insulin resistance impairs this process. Normally, insulin helps the liver efficiently break down and convert fats. However, in insulin-resistant individuals, the liver's ability to oxidize (break down) fatty acids is compromised, leading to fat accumulation in liver tissue and inflammation. This results in **non-alcoholic steatohepatitis (NASH)**, a more advanced and potentially more dangerous form of fatty liver disease.
- **Inflammation and Fibrosis**: Over time, the fat accumulation and insulin resistance trigger an inflammatory response in the liver. This inflammation, combined with oxidative stress, can lead to liver cell damage and fibrosis (scarring of the liver tissue). If left unchecked, this can progress to cirrhosis, liver failure, and even liver cancer.

3. The Role of Insulin Resistance in the Development of Type 2 Diabetes

The link between insulin resistance and **type 2 diabetes** is well-documented. Insulin resistance is a primary underlying factor in the development of diabetes, as it impairs the body's ability to regulate blood sugar levels effectively.

How Insulin Resistance Leads to Type 2 Diabetes:

- **Impaired Glucose Uptake**: In people with insulin resistance, muscle, fat, and liver cells do not respond as

effectively to insulin. As a result, glucose remains in the bloodstream rather than being absorbed into cells for energy. The pancreas compensates by releasing more insulin to help cells take up glucose. However, over time, the pancreas can become unable to produce enough insulin to keep up with the body's demands, leading to **hyperglycemia** (high blood sugar).
- **Elevated Blood Sugar Levels**: As blood sugar levels remain elevated, the liver continues to produce glucose, exacerbating the problem. This creates a vicious cycle where both insulin resistance and high blood sugar levels reinforce each other. Over time, the body becomes unable to maintain normal blood sugar levels, and **type 2 diabetes** develops.
- **Beta-Cell Dysfunction**: The pancreas produces insulin through specialized cells called **beta cells**. In the early stages of insulin resistance, the pancreas compensates by producing more insulin. However, chronic insulin resistance leads to beta-cell dysfunction, where the pancreas can no longer produce sufficient amounts of insulin. This inability to produce enough insulin to overcome the body's insulin resistance is a key factor in the onset of type 2 diabetes.
- **Increased Risk of Cardiovascular Disease**: Both insulin resistance and type 2 diabetes are associated with an increased risk of cardiovascular disease (CVD). Elevated blood sugar levels and high insulin levels contribute to **vascular inflammation**, damage to blood vessels, and the buildup of plaque in the arteries (atherosclerosis), all of which increase the risk of heart attack and stroke.

4. The Bi-Directional Relationship Between Insulin Resistance, Fatty Liver, and Diabetes

The relationship between insulin resistance, fatty liver, and type 2 diabetes is bi-directional, meaning that each condition can exacerbate the other, creating a vicious cycle that is difficult to break.

How Fatty Liver Exacerbates Insulin Resistance:

- **Liver Dysfunction**: In individuals with fatty liver, the liver's ability to regulate glucose and fat metabolism is impaired, which makes insulin resistance worse. The liver becomes less sensitive to insulin, leading to higher blood sugar levels and the release of excess glucose into the bloodstream. This worsens insulin resistance and contributes to the development of type 2 diabetes.
- **Increased Inflammation**: Fatty liver disease triggers inflammation in the liver and throughout the body. Chronic inflammation is a key factor in the development of both insulin resistance and diabetes. The liver's inflammatory response contributes to further impairment of insulin signaling, making it harder for the body to use insulin effectively.
- **Fatty Liver as a Marker for Insulin Resistance**: Studies have shown that the presence of fatty liver disease is often an early indicator of insulin resistance and can predict the development of type 2 diabetes. People with NAFLD or NASH are at a higher risk of developing diabetes, even if they do not have the condition initially.

How Insulin Resistance Exacerbates Fatty Liver Disease:

- **Increased Fat Accumulation**: As mentioned earlier, insulin resistance leads to the increased release of free fatty acids from adipose tissue. These fatty acids are delivered to the liver, where they are stored as fat. This contributes to the development of fatty liver disease.
- **Impaired Liver Function**: Insulin resistance hampers the liver's ability to process glucose and fats efficiently, leading to increased fat storage, liver cell damage, and eventual progression to NASH and cirrhosis.

5. Managing Insulin Resistance to Improve Liver Health

Given the strong link between insulin resistance, fatty liver, and type 2 diabetes, managing insulin resistance is crucial for improving liver health and reducing the risk of diabetes. Here are key strategies for managing insulin resistance:

- **Healthy Eating**: A balanced diet rich in **fiber, healthy fats**, and **antioxidants** can improve insulin sensitivity. Avoiding refined sugars, processed foods, and excessive carbohydrates is essential to maintaining stable blood sugar levels and reducing insulin resistance.
- **Regular Exercise**: Physical activity is one of the most effective ways to improve insulin sensitivity. Exercise helps muscles use glucose more effectively, which reduces the amount of insulin needed by the body. It also helps burn excess fat, which is crucial for reducing liver fat accumulation.

- **Weight Management**: Maintaining a healthy weight is critical for improving insulin resistance. Even a modest weight loss (5-10% of body weight) can significantly improve insulin sensitivity and reduce liver fat.
- **Medications**: In some cases, medications such as **metformin** may be prescribed to help manage insulin resistance. These medications can improve the body's response to insulin and help regulate blood sugar levels.

The Importance of Weight Loss and How It Helps Your Liver

Weight loss plays a pivotal role in managing and potentially reversing fatty liver disease, particularly **non-alcoholic fatty liver disease (NAFLD)** and **non-alcoholic steatohepatitis (NASH)**. Both of these conditions are strongly associated with obesity and excess body fat, especially around the abdominal area. When you lose weight, you can significantly reduce fat accumulation in the liver, improve liver function, and prevent further damage. However, not all weight loss approaches are equally effective or safe, so it's crucial to understand why **gradual, sustainable weight loss** is key to supporting liver health.

1. How Excess Weight Affects the Liver

Before delving into the specifics of weight loss, it's important to understand why excess weight is so damaging to liver health.

Fat Accumulation in the Liver

Excessive body fat, particularly visceral fat (fat stored around the organs), contributes directly to fat accumulation in the liver. When the liver becomes overwhelmed by fat deposits, it results in **fatty liver disease**, which, if left untreated, can lead to **inflammation**, **liver fibrosis**, and, in severe cases, cirrhosis.

Inflammation and Insulin Resistance

Obesity also increases the release of **inflammatory cytokines**, which promote inflammation in the liver. Chronic low-grade inflammation contributes to **insulin resistance**, which is a critical factor in the progression of fatty liver disease. This results in further fat storage in the liver, creating a vicious cycle that worsens liver function over time.

Increased Risk of Other Health Issues

Obesity, especially abdominal fat, is also linked to **high blood pressure**, **high cholesterol**, and **diabetes**, all of which further increase the risk of liver damage. When combined with fatty liver disease, these conditions increase the overall burden on the liver, making weight loss even more crucial.

2. Why Gradual, Sustainable Weight Loss Is Crucial for Liver Health

While weight loss is beneficial, how you lose the weight matters. Rapid weight loss, especially through fad diets or extreme measures, can actually **worsen liver function** in some cases. Here's why **gradual, sustainable weight loss** is the most effective approach:

A. Preventing Fatty Liver from Worsening

Rapid weight loss—such as losing large amounts of weight in a short period of time—can cause the liver to release fat too quickly into the bloodstream. This sudden influx of fat can overwhelm the liver and worsen **fatty liver disease**. This is particularly risky for individuals with NASH, as it can trigger **liver inflammation** and further damage liver cells.

Gradual weight loss, on the other hand, allows the liver to adjust to the changes more effectively. The liver can metabolize and eliminate fat at a more controlled rate, reducing the likelihood of complications such as liver inflammation or scarring.

B. Supporting Metabolic Processes

Losing weight too quickly can also disrupt metabolic processes. The body needs time to adjust to changes in diet and physical activity, and rapid weight loss can stress the body, leading to **muscle loss** and a **slower metabolism**. This can make it harder to maintain weight loss in the long run, leading to the **yo-yo effect**, where lost weight is regained quickly.

A gradual, sustainable approach allows the body to preserve lean muscle mass, maintain metabolic function, and keep the weight off in the long term. It also reduces the risk of **nutrient deficiencies** that can arise from crash diets, ensuring the liver receives the proper nutrients it needs for optimal function.

C. Reducing Inflammation and Insulin Resistance

Gradual weight loss has been shown to have a positive effect on **insulin sensitivity** and **inflammation**. When fat is reduced at a controlled pace, the body has the opportunity to improve its ability to respond to insulin, which helps reduce fat accumulation in the liver. Additionally, reducing visceral fat gradually lowers the levels of inflammatory markers in the body, helping to reverse liver damage and prevent further progression of fatty liver disease.

D. Long-Term Liver Protection

Sustainable weight loss doesn't just shrink the size of your liver; it can reverse the **biochemical processes** that cause liver damage in the first place. As you lose weight at a sustainable pace, you reduce fat deposits, lower liver enzyme levels, and improve **liver function tests**. Over time, this can significantly reduce the risk of developing more severe liver conditions, such as cirrhosis or liver cancer.

3. The Science of Gradual Weight Loss

The optimal rate of weight loss for liver health is generally around **1 to 2 pounds (0.5 to 1 kg) per week**. This amount of weight loss is considered safe and effective for long-term health. Research indicates that this gradual rate allows for the following benefits:

- **Fat Loss without Muscle Loss**: Gradual weight loss prioritizes fat loss over muscle loss, preserving lean muscle tissue, which is crucial for maintaining a healthy

metabolism. Muscle tissue helps to burn calories, and retaining it ensures that you don't stall your progress once the weight loss slows down.
- **Improved Liver Fat Content**: Studies have shown that losing just **5-10% of your body weight** can lead to a significant reduction in liver fat, even in people with advanced fatty liver disease. Gradual weight loss helps ensure that this reduction in liver fat happens over time, allowing the liver to adjust without excessive strain.
- **Sustained Insulin Sensitivity**: Gradual weight loss helps improve **insulin sensitivity**, which is a critical factor in reversing insulin resistance and preventing the progression of type 2 diabetes. Insulin sensitivity helps the liver better regulate blood sugar and fat storage, reducing the chances of fat buildup in the liver.
- **Reduced Risk of Gallstones**: Rapid weight loss is associated with an increased risk of developing **gallstones**, which can be harmful to the liver. Gradual weight loss helps minimize this risk, ensuring that the liver and gallbladder function properly as you shed pounds.

4. The Best Approaches to Gradual, Sustainable Weight Loss

Now that we understand why gradual weight loss is so important for liver health, let's explore how to achieve it through sustainable methods:

A. Diet Modification

The foundation of any effective weight loss plan starts with a healthy diet. Focusing on **whole foods**—such as vegetables, fruits, lean proteins, healthy fats (e.g., omega-3 fatty acids), and high-fiber carbohydrates—can promote weight loss while providing essential nutrients for liver health. Avoiding refined sugars, processed foods, and trans fats is crucial for reducing inflammation and fat accumulation in the liver.

Key dietary strategies:

- Incorporate foods rich in antioxidants, such as berries, spinach, and nuts, to reduce liver inflammation.
- Focus on **omega-3 fatty acids** found in fish like salmon, walnuts, and flaxseeds, which help reduce liver fat.
- Increase your intake of **fiber-rich foods**, like whole grains, legumes, and vegetables, which help improve digestion and support liver detoxification.

B. Regular Exercise

Exercise is essential for supporting sustainable weight loss. Combining **aerobic exercise** (like walking, jogging, or swimming) with **strength training** (such as weight lifting or bodyweight exercises) helps you burn fat, preserve muscle mass, and boost metabolism.

Exercise recommendations:

- Aim for at least **150 minutes per week** of moderate-intensity aerobic activity (or 75 minutes of vigorous-intensity activity).

- Include **strength training exercises** at least two days per week to build muscle and support weight loss.

C. Behavioral and Lifestyle Changes

Sustainable weight loss requires more than just dieting and exercising; it also involves making lasting lifestyle changes. This can include:

- Getting adequate **sleep** (7-9 hours per night), as poor sleep is linked to weight gain and metabolic dysfunction.
- **Managing stress** through techniques such as mindfulness, yoga, or meditation, as chronic stress can increase the likelihood of overeating and weight gain.
- **Setting realistic goals** and tracking progress, focusing on small, achievable milestones that encourage long-term success.

Chapter 3: The Ideal Fatty Liver Diet – A 7-Day Meal Plan to Get You Started

A healthy, balanced diet is one of the most powerful tools in combating fatty liver disease. Whether you have **non-alcoholic fatty liver disease (NAFLD)** or **non-alcoholic steatohepatitis (NASH)**, nutrition plays a vital role in reversing liver damage, reducing fat accumulation, and supporting overall liver function. The key to a liver-friendly diet lies in choosing nutrient-dense, anti-inflammatory foods that promote liver health while avoiding foods that can exacerbate fat storage and inflammation.

In this chapter, we will explore the **ideal fatty liver diet** and provide you with a **7-day meal plan** to help you get started on your journey toward healing and better liver health.

1. Core Principles of the Fatty Liver Diet

Before diving into the meal plan, it's important to understand the principles behind the diet. These principles focus on nourishing your liver, reducing fat, and addressing insulin resistance.

- **High in Fiber**: Fiber-rich foods help promote digestion, regulate blood sugar levels, and reduce liver fat. Foods like fruits, vegetables, legumes, and whole grains are essential.
- **Rich in Antioxidants**: Antioxidants protect the liver from oxidative stress, which contributes to liver damage. Foods like berries, leafy greens, nuts, and seeds are loaded with antioxidants.

- **Healthy Fats**: Healthy fats, especially **omega-3 fatty acids**, reduce liver fat and inflammation. Sources include fatty fish (like salmon), olive oil, and flaxseeds.
- **Lean Protein**: Protein helps preserve muscle mass and aids in fat loss. Opt for lean proteins like chicken breast, turkey, tofu, and legumes.
- **Low in Refined Carbs and Sugars**: Refined carbohydrates (white bread, pastries) and added sugars can increase fat accumulation in the liver. Reducing these foods helps lower insulin resistance and improve liver function.
- **Anti-Inflammatory**: Chronic inflammation is a significant contributor to fatty liver disease. Including anti-inflammatory foods like turmeric, ginger, and green tea can help manage inflammation.

2. What to Avoid on the Fatty Liver Diet

Certain foods and beverages can worsen fatty liver disease or slow its reversal. These include:

- **Sugary Beverages**: Soda, sweetened coffee, and energy drinks are high in sugar and can contribute to fat buildup in the liver.
- **Processed Foods**: Highly processed foods, such as fast food, chips, and ready-to-eat snacks, are high in unhealthy fats and refined sugars.
- **Alcohol**: Even though your fatty liver may not be alcohol-induced, alcohol can further damage your liver and exacerbate fat accumulation.

- **Trans Fats**: Found in many packaged snacks, baked goods, and fried foods, trans fats increase liver fat and inflammation.
- **Refined Carbohydrates**: Foods like white bread, pasta, and pastries can spike blood sugar levels and lead to insulin resistance, worsening fatty liver disease.

3. The 7-Day Fatty Liver Meal Plan

This 7-day meal plan is designed to provide balanced, liver-friendly meals that promote fat loss, reduce inflammation, and improve liver function. The plan includes whole, natural foods that are rich in antioxidants, healthy fats, and fiber. Portions can be adjusted based on your individual needs, but the goal is to create a sustainable, healthy eating pattern that you can maintain beyond the initial week.

Day 1: Kickstart with Fiber and Omega-3s

Breakfast:

- **Overnight Oats with Chia Seeds and Berries**: Rolled oats, chia seeds, almond milk, and fresh berries (blueberries, strawberries). Top with a handful of walnuts for an added omega-3 boost.
- **Green Tea**: A cup of green tea to increase antioxidant intake and improve fat metabolism.

Lunch:

- **Grilled Salmon Salad**: Grilled salmon on a bed of mixed greens (spinach, kale), cucumber, avocado, and cherry tomatoes, with a lemon-olive oil dressing.
- **Whole Grain Roll**: A small serving of whole-grain bread for fiber.

Snack:

- **Apple with Almond Butter**: A fresh apple paired with a tablespoon of almond butter for a dose of healthy fats and fiber.

Dinner:

- **Quinoa and Veggie Stir-Fry**: Cooked quinoa with sautéed vegetables like broccoli, bell peppers, and zucchini, drizzled with olive oil. Add a sprinkle of turmeric for its anti-inflammatory properties.
- **Lemon Water**: To help with digestion and detoxification.

Day 2: Focus on Lean Protein and Antioxidants

Breakfast:

- **Greek Yogurt with Walnuts and Berries**: Full-fat, plain Greek yogurt topped with fresh berries, chia seeds, and chopped walnuts. Greek yogurt is a great source of protein and probiotics.
- **Black Coffee or Herbal Tea**: Drink coffee in moderation or opt for herbal tea.

Lunch:

- **Turkey and Avocado Wrap**: Whole grain wrap filled with lean turkey breast, sliced avocado, spinach, and mustard or hummus for flavor.
- **Carrot Sticks with Hummus**: A serving of fresh carrots with homemade hummus for extra fiber and healthy fats.

Snack:

- **Cucumber and Tomato Salad**: Chopped cucumber, tomatoes, and red onion, drizzled with olive oil and a splash of apple cider vinegar.

Dinner:

- **Grilled Chicken with Roasted Brussels Sprouts**: Skinless grilled chicken breast paired with roasted Brussels sprouts and sweet potato.
- **Herbal Tea**: A calming cup of herbal tea to finish the day.

Day 3: Boost Fiber with Legumes and Vegetables

Breakfast:

- **Smoothie with Spinach, Banana, and Flaxseeds**: A smoothie made with spinach, a banana, flaxseeds, almond milk, and a scoop of protein powder (optional).
- **Water with Lemon**: A glass of water with lemon to kickstart your day.

Lunch:

- **Lentil Soup**: Homemade lentil soup with carrots, celery, onions, and garlic. Lentils are rich in fiber and protein, making them perfect for liver health.
- **Side of Mixed Greens**: A small side salad with olive oil and vinegar dressing.

Snack:

- **Cottage Cheese with Berries**: A serving of cottage cheese paired with a handful of fresh berries.

Dinner:

- **Baked Cod with Roasted Vegetables**: Cod fillets baked with lemon and herbs, served with roasted root vegetables like sweet potatoes and carrots.
- **Water or Green Tea**: Stay hydrated and enjoy a warm cup of green tea.

Day 4: Heart-Healthy Fats and Whole Grains

Breakfast:

- **Chia Pudding with Coconut and Almonds**: Chia seeds soaked in almond milk, topped with coconut flakes, sliced almonds, and a handful of berries.
- **Green Tea**: For added antioxidants.

Lunch:

- **Chickpea and Spinach Salad**: A hearty salad with chickpeas, spinach, cucumbers, tomatoes, red onion, and a tahini dressing.

- **Whole Wheat Pita Bread**: A small portion of whole wheat pita for extra fiber.

Snack:

- **Carrot and Celery Sticks with Guacamole**: A healthy snack of raw veggies paired with guacamole for a dose of healthy fats.

Dinner:

- **Grilled Tofu with Stir-Fried Vegetables**: Tofu grilled or pan-fried, paired with stir-fried vegetables like bell peppers, broccoli, and snap peas.
- **Water**: Keep hydrated throughout the evening.

Day 5: High in Omega-3s and Antioxidants

Breakfast:

- **Avocado Toast with Eggs**: Whole grain toast topped with mashed avocado, a poached egg, and a sprinkle of chia seeds.
- **Green Tea**: A perfect morning pick-me-up.

Lunch:

- **Salmon and Avocado Bowl**: A bowl with grilled salmon, avocado, cucumber, mixed greens, and a drizzle of olive oil and lemon.
- **Steamed Asparagus**: Steamed asparagus as a side for extra fiber and antioxidants.

Snack:

- **Mixed Nuts:** A handful of mixed nuts (almonds, walnuts, pecans) for healthy fats and protein.

Dinner:

- **Baked Chicken with Quinoa and Kale:** Skinless baked chicken breast served with quinoa and sautéed kale.
- **Herbal Tea:** A calming, digestive-friendly tea to end your day.

Day 6: Healing Herbs and Plant-Based Proteins

Breakfast:

- **Turmeric Smoothie:** A smoothie made with coconut milk, banana, turmeric, spinach, and ginger. Turmeric is a powerful anti-inflammatory herb.
- **Black Coffee:** A small cup of black coffee if desired.

Lunch:

- **Grilled Veggie Wrap:** A whole grain wrap with grilled vegetables (eggplant, zucchini, peppers), hummus, and spinach.
- **Side Salad:** A mixed green salad with olive oil and balsamic vinegar dressing.

Snack:

- **Berries with Almonds:** A handful of fresh berries paired with raw almonds.

Dinner:

- **Tofu Stir-Fry with Brown Rice**: Tofu, bell peppers, and broccoli stir-fried in olive oil, served over brown rice.
- **Water with Lemon**: Hydration is key to support liver detoxification.

Day 7: Balanced Meal with Lean Protein and Healthy Fats

Breakfast:

- **Omelette with Veggies and Feta**: An omelette with spinach, tomatoes, mushrooms, and a sprinkle of feta cheese.
- **Herbal Tea**: A soothing tea to start the day.

Lunch:

- **Grilled Chicken Salad with Quinoa**: Grilled chicken breast on top of quinoa, mixed greens, avocado, and cucumber, dressed with olive oil and lemon.
- **Fruit**: A small serving of fresh fruit like an apple or orange.

Snack:

- **Cucumber and Hummus**: Fresh cucumber slices served with hummus for a light, satisfying snack.

Dinner:

- **Grilled Salmon with Sweet Potato**: Salmon fillet grilled with herbs and lemon, paired with roasted sweet potato and steamed broccoli.
- **Lemon Water**: To help with digestion and liver cleansing.

4. Tips for Success on the Fatty Liver Diet

- **Stay Consistent**: A healthy, liver-friendly diet works best when you stick with it. Avoid frequent cheat meals or processed foods.
- **Hydrate Well**: Drink plenty of water throughout the day to support detoxification and liver function.
- **Small, Frequent Meals**: Eating smaller, balanced meals every 3–4 hours helps maintain stable blood sugar levels and supports liver health.
- **Physical Activity**: Combine your diet with regular physical activity, such as walking, cycling, or strength training, to help reduce liver fat and improve insulin sensitivity.

By following this 7-day meal plan, you'll be on your way to improving liver function and reducing fat accumulation. It's just the start of a healthy lifestyle that will support your liver for years to come.

Day-by-Day Guide: A Structured Plan to Jump-Start a Liver-Healthy Lifestyle with Easy-to-Follow Meals

Adopting a liver-healthy lifestyle can feel overwhelming at first, especially when dealing with the complexities of fatty liver disease. However, with a structured plan, it becomes easier to incorporate liver-supportive foods into your daily routine. This day-by-day guide offers a simple, balanced approach to jump-starting your liver-healing journey with easy-to-follow meals that nourish, detoxify, and heal the liver. Each day includes liver-friendly recipes that support detoxification, reduce fat accumulation, and boost overall liver function.

Day 1: Cleanse and Energize with Antioxidants

Focus for the Day: Antioxidants and healthy fats to help combat oxidative stress and start the detox process.

Breakfast: Green Detox Smoothie

Start your day with a smoothie packed with green vegetables, fiber, and healthy fats to support liver detox. This smoothie is rich in antioxidants and vitamins, which help to neutralize free radicals and reduce inflammation in the liver.

Ingredients:

- 1 cup spinach
- 1/2 avocado
- 1/2 banana
- 1 tbsp flaxseeds (ground)
- 1 tbsp chia seeds
- 1/2 cup unsweetened almond milk
- 1/2 cup coconut water
- 1 tsp spirulina (optional, for added detoxification)
- Ice cubes

Instructions:

1. Combine all ingredients in a blender.
2. Blend until smooth, adding more water or almond milk if needed to reach desired consistency.
3. Pour into a glass and enjoy!

Why it's good for your liver: Spinach is a rich source of antioxidants, while avocado provides healthy fats that support liver function. The chia and flaxseeds provide fiber, which helps remove toxins from the body.

Lunch: Grilled Salmon and Kale Salad

Packed with healthy omega-3 fatty acids and fiber, this salmon and kale salad is an ideal meal to support liver detox and reduce inflammation.

Ingredients:

- 1 salmon fillet
- 2 cups kale (massaged with olive oil)
- 1/2 cup quinoa (cooked)
- 1/2 avocado, sliced
- 1/4 cup cherry tomatoes, halved
- 1 tbsp olive oil (for dressing)
- 1 tbsp lemon juice
- Salt and pepper to taste

Instructions:

1. Season the salmon fillet with olive oil, salt, and pepper.

2. Grill or bake the salmon at 400°F for 12–15 minutes, or until cooked through.
3. In a large bowl, massage the kale with a bit of olive oil and salt until it softens.
4. Add quinoa, avocado, cherry tomatoes, and grilled salmon to the kale.
5. Drizzle with olive oil and lemon juice, toss, and serve.

Why it's good for your liver: Salmon is an excellent source of omega-3 fatty acids, which reduce liver fat. Kale is a detoxifying vegetable high in fiber and antioxidants, which support liver function and reduce oxidative stress.

Snack: Fresh Carrot Sticks with Hummus

A simple, fiber-rich snack that helps reduce fat in the liver and maintain energy levels throughout the day.

Ingredients:

- 2 medium carrots, peeled and cut into sticks
- 2 tbsp hummus (store-bought or homemade)

Instructions:

1. Cut carrots into sticks.
2. Serve with hummus for dipping.

Why it's good for your liver: Carrots are high in beta-carotene, which helps reduce liver inflammation. Hummus provides healthy fats and protein to keep you satisfied between meals.

Dinner: Sweet Potato and Lentil Stew

This hearty, fiber-rich stew supports liver health with its anti-inflammatory properties and high fiber content. Sweet potatoes are rich in beta-carotene, which helps cleanse the liver.

Ingredients:

- 1 medium sweet potato, peeled and cubed
- 1/2 cup dry lentils (rinsed)
- 1 can (14 oz) diced tomatoes
- 1 onion, chopped
- 2 cloves garlic, minced
- 1 tsp turmeric
- 1/2 tsp cumin
- 1/2 tsp smoked paprika
- 1 tbsp olive oil
- 4 cups vegetable broth
- Salt and pepper to taste
- Fresh cilantro for garnish

Instructions:

1. In a large pot, heat olive oil over medium heat. Add onions and garlic, and sauté until softened.
2. Add the turmeric, cumin, and smoked paprika, and stir for 1 minute.
3. Add the sweet potatoes, lentils, diced tomatoes, and vegetable broth.
4. Bring to a boil, then reduce heat and simmer for 30–40 minutes, until lentils and sweet potatoes are tender.

5. Season with salt and pepper, and garnish with fresh cilantro before serving.

Why it's good for your liver: Sweet potatoes are rich in antioxidants and fiber, while lentils provide plant-based protein and support digestion. Turmeric has potent anti-inflammatory properties, which reduce liver stress.

Day 2: Boosting Liver Function with Fiber and Protein

Focus for the Day: Emphasizing fiber and lean protein to support liver repair and help with fat loss.

Breakfast: Oats with Berries and Chia Seeds

A fiber-packed breakfast to jump-start the day and improve liver function. Oats are rich in beta-glucans, which help to regulate cholesterol and liver fat.

Ingredients:

- 1/2 cup rolled oats
- 1 cup water or almond milk
- 1 tbsp chia seeds
- 1/2 cup mixed berries (blueberries, raspberries, strawberries)
- 1 tsp cinnamon
- 1 tbsp almond butter (optional)

Instructions:

1. Cook the oats according to package instructions using water or almond milk.
2. Stir in chia seeds, cinnamon, and almond butter (if using).
3. Top with mixed berries before serving.

Why it's good for your liver: Oats are high in fiber, which supports digestion and liver health. Berries are rich in antioxidants, and chia seeds provide omega-3 fatty acids.

Lunch: Quinoa and Chickpea Salad

This plant-based salad is full of fiber, protein, and healthy fats. It helps support liver detox and provides steady energy throughout the day.

Ingredients:

- 1 cup cooked quinoa
- 1/2 cup chickpeas (cooked or canned)
- 1/2 cucumber, diced
- 1/4 red onion, thinly sliced
- 1 tbsp olive oil
- 1 tbsp lemon juice
- Fresh parsley, chopped
- Salt and pepper to taste

Instructions:

1. In a large bowl, combine the quinoa, chickpeas, cucumber, red onion, and parsley.
2. Drizzle with olive oil and lemon juice, and toss to combine.

3. Season with salt and pepper to taste.

Why it's good for your liver: Chickpeas are an excellent source of fiber and protein, which help stabilize blood sugar levels and improve liver function. Quinoa is rich in magnesium, a mineral that supports detoxification.

Snack: Apple with Walnuts

A healthy snack that combines the benefits of fiber and healthy fats to keep your liver and energy levels balanced.

Ingredients:

- 1 medium apple, sliced
- A handful of raw walnuts

Instructions:

1. Slice the apple and pair it with walnuts for a simple snack.

Why it's good for your liver: Apples are high in fiber and antioxidants, while walnuts provide omega-3 fatty acids that help reduce inflammation in the liver.

Dinner: Grilled Chicken with Roasted Vegetables

A simple, protein-rich dinner with healthy fats and fiber to support liver healing.

Ingredients:

- 1 chicken breast (skinless)
- 1 zucchini, sliced
- 1 red bell pepper, chopped
- 1 sweet potato, cubed
- 2 tbsp olive oil
- 1 tsp rosemary
- Salt and pepper to taste

Instructions:

1. Preheat the oven to 400°F (200°C).
2. Toss the vegetables with olive oil, rosemary, salt, and pepper, and roast in the oven for 25–30 minutes until tender.
3. While the vegetables are roasting, grill or bake the chicken breast for 15–20 minutes, or until fully cooked.
4. Serve the chicken alongside the roasted vegetables.

Why it's good for your liver: Chicken is a lean source of protein, while sweet potatoes provide fiber and antioxidants. The healthy fats from olive oil help reduce liver fat.

Tips for Success

- **Hydrate**: Drink plenty of water throughout the day to aid in digestion and liver detoxification.
- **Keep Meals Simple**: Focus on whole, unprocessed foods and avoid overcomplicating meals.
- **Listen to Your Body**: Pay attention to how you feel after each meal to adjust portion sizes or ingredients for optimal liver health.

The Power of Portion Control and Meal Timing: Tips on Portion Sizes and When to Eat for Optimal Liver Health

When it comes to managing fatty liver disease and supporting the healing of your liver, portion control and meal timing are two of the most impactful factors you can incorporate into your daily routine. Both are vital elements of a well-balanced, liver-healthy diet that help regulate blood sugar levels, prevent overeating, reduce fat accumulation in the liver, and promote overall wellness.

Why Portion Control Matters for Liver Health

Portion control plays a critical role in managing liver health, especially for individuals with fatty liver disease (NAFLD or NASH). Excess calorie consumption, particularly from processed foods, unhealthy fats, and sugary snacks, contributes to fat buildup in the liver and exacerbates the condition. When you practice portion control, you can avoid overeating, regulate your calorie intake, and ensure that your body is getting the right amount of nutrients to support liver function without overloading it.

How Portion Control Impacts Fatty Liver Disease

1. **Prevents Overload on the Liver**: The liver is responsible for processing and metabolizing fats, carbohydrates, and proteins. Overeating, especially foods high in unhealthy fats or refined sugars, puts extra strain on the liver, increasing fat accumulation and impairing liver function. By controlling portion

sizes, you give your liver the time and capacity to process nutrients properly without becoming overburdened.
2. **Helps with Weight Management**: Maintaining a healthy weight is one of the most effective ways to manage and even reverse fatty liver disease. Portion control helps prevent weight gain and encourages gradual, sustainable weight loss by allowing you to eat foods in appropriate amounts that support metabolism and liver detoxification without excess calorie intake.
3. **Regulates Blood Sugar**: A critical factor in managing fatty liver is controlling blood sugar levels. High blood sugar spikes can worsen insulin resistance, which is linked to fatty liver disease. By controlling portion sizes, especially with carbohydrates, you can stabilize blood sugar levels and reduce insulin spikes, which can help prevent further liver damage.

Tips for Portion Control to Promote Liver Health

1. Use Smaller Plates and Bowls One of the easiest ways to control portion sizes is to serve your meals on smaller plates and bowls. This trick works by tricking your brain into thinking you're eating more than you actually are. The size of your plate can influence how much food you feel compelled to put on it, and smaller plates help you eat less while still feeling satisfied.

2. Focus on Balanced Meals When preparing meals, make sure each plate consists of healthy portions of lean protein, fiber-rich vegetables, and whole grains. A good rule of thumb is to fill half your plate with vegetables, a quarter with lean protein (such as fish, chicken, or legumes), and a quarter with whole grains or healthy starches like sweet potatoes or quinoa. This ensures you're consuming a variety of nutrients, helping your liver work optimally.

3. Learn About Serving Sizes To avoid overeating, it's essential to understand what constitutes a proper portion size. A serving of lean protein (like fish or chicken) is about the size of the palm of your hand, while a serving of grains or starches (such as quinoa or rice) is about the size of your fist. For vegetables, you can typically aim to fill half of your plate with non-starchy veggies like spinach, kale, or broccoli.

4. Eat More Fiber-Rich Foods Fiber is crucial for liver health because it helps bind and remove toxins from the digestive system, reducing the strain on the liver. Aim to fill half of your plate with non-starchy vegetables and high-fiber fruits like berries and apples. Fiber also keeps you feeling fuller for longer, making portion control easier to maintain.

5. Avoid Overeating by Eating Slowly It takes about 20 minutes for your brain to signal that you're full. Eating too quickly can lead to overeating and cause you to exceed the amount of food your liver can efficiently process. Slow down, chew your food thoroughly, and savor each bite. This practice helps prevent overeating and promotes better digestion.

6. Limit High-Calorie, Low-Nutrient Foods Refined sugars, processed snacks, and fried foods are high in calories but offer little in terms of nutrients. These foods contribute to fat accumulation in the liver and can exacerbate liver damage. Instead, focus on whole, nutrient-dense foods that support liver function, such as leafy greens, lean proteins, healthy fats, and whole grains.

Meal Timing: When to Eat for Optimal Liver Health

Meal timing is just as important as portion control when it comes to maintaining liver health. The timing of your meals can impact how well your liver processes nutrients, how efficiently your body metabolizes fats, and even how you maintain stable blood sugar levels throughout the day.

1. Eat Breakfast Within an Hour of Waking Starting your day with a balanced breakfast within an hour of waking up is essential for maintaining stable blood sugar levels and preventing liver overload. Breakfast jump-starts your metabolism and provides your liver with nutrients for detoxification and energy. Choose liver-friendly breakfast options such as oatmeal with chia seeds, a green smoothie, or scrambled eggs with spinach and avocado.

2. Space Your Meals Throughout the Day Instead of eating large, heavy meals that can overwhelm your digestive system and liver, aim for three balanced meals with 1–2 healthy snacks spaced throughout the day. This strategy helps maintain stable blood sugar levels, reduces the risk of insulin resistance, and allows your liver enough time to process the food you've eaten.

3. Avoid Late-Night Snacking Late-night eating, especially when consuming high-calorie or sugary foods, can contribute to insulin resistance and disrupt your liver's detoxification process. The liver is most effective at detoxing during sleep, and eating too close to bedtime can interfere with this process. Aim to finish your last meal or snack at least 2–3 hours before bed to allow your liver time to focus on repair and detoxification while you sleep.

4. Consider Intermittent Fasting Intermittent fasting (IF) has gained popularity for its potential benefits to liver health, particularly in reducing insulin resistance and promoting fat metabolism. With intermittent fasting, you restrict your eating window to a specific period (e.g., 8 hours) and fast for the remaining 16 hours of the day. This gives the liver time to focus on detoxification and repair, reducing fat accumulation and promoting a healthier liver. However, it's important to consult with a healthcare provider before beginning any fasting regimen.

5. Avoid Overloading on Carbs at One Meal Large amounts of carbohydrates, particularly from refined sugars and processed grains, can spike insulin levels and exacerbate fatty liver disease. Instead of loading up on carbs at a single meal, spread them out over the day. Focus on whole, complex carbohydrates such as sweet potatoes, quinoa, and brown rice, which are easier for the liver to process and metabolize.

Benefits of Proper Portion Control and Meal Timing for Liver Health

- **Reduces Fatty Liver Accumulation**: By managing portion sizes and meal timing, you can prevent excessive calorie consumption and fat buildup in the liver, a key factor in the progression of fatty liver disease.

- **Improves Metabolism**: Consistent meal timing supports a steady metabolism, which allows your liver to process nutrients more efficiently, reducing the likelihood of insulin resistance.
- **Promotes Weight Loss**: Portion control helps with weight management, and maintaining a healthy weight reduces the risk of further liver damage and promotes healing.
- **Supports Detoxification**: Spacing meals throughout the day and giving your liver ample time to rest and detoxify during fasting periods helps the liver remove toxins and perform essential repairs.

Incorporating Intermittent Fasting: Exploring the Potential Benefits for Fatty Liver Disease

Intermittent fasting (IF) has become increasingly popular in recent years for its potential to support weight loss, improve metabolic health, and provide numerous benefits for overall well-being. Among its many advantages, one of the most promising is its ability to help manage and even reverse fatty liver disease (NAFLD and NASH). In this section, we'll explore the science behind intermittent fasting, its potential benefits for liver health, and how to incorporate this practice into your daily life.

What is Intermittent Fasting?

Intermittent fasting is an eating pattern that alternates between periods of fasting (no food or calorie intake) and eating. Rather than focusing on what you eat, intermittent fasting focuses on when you eat, cycling between eating windows and fasting periods. There are several common methods of intermittent fasting, such as:

- **The 16/8 Method**: This involves fasting for 16 hours and eating all meals within an 8-hour window. For example, you might eat from noon to 8 PM and fast from 8 PM to noon the next day.
- **The 5:2 Diet**: In this method, you eat normally for five days of the week and restrict calorie intake to about 500-600 calories on the other two non-consecutive days.
- **Alternate-Day Fasting**: This method involves alternating between fasting days (consuming very few or no calories) and eating days.

While intermittent fasting is not a diet in the traditional sense, it is a structured approach to eating that focuses on reducing overall calorie intake while also providing specific windows for the body to rest, repair, and heal.

The Science Behind Intermittent Fasting and Fatty Liver Disease

The key to understanding the potential benefits of intermittent fasting for fatty liver disease lies in the physiological changes that occur during fasting periods. When you fast, your body shifts from using glucose (sugar) as its primary energy source to using fat stores for fuel. This metabolic shift helps the body burn fat, and in the case of fatty liver disease, it can specifically target liver fat. Here's how intermittent fasting may help:

1. Reduction in Insulin Resistance

Insulin resistance is a primary driver of fatty liver disease. In this condition, the liver becomes less responsive to insulin, a hormone that regulates blood sugar. This results in elevated blood sugar and increased fat storage in the liver.

Intermittent fasting helps improve insulin sensitivity by reducing the constant influx of glucose and insulin that occurs with frequent meals. During fasting periods, insulin levels drop, and the liver's ability to process fat and metabolize glucose improves. By improving insulin sensitivity, intermittent fasting can help reduce the accumulation of fat in the liver and improve liver function.

2. Promotion of Fat Burning and Liver Detoxification

Fasting induces a process called **lipolysis**, where the body breaks down stored fat into fatty acids and glycerol, which can then be used for energy. This process helps reduce fat deposits in the liver, particularly harmful visceral fat (the fat surrounding organs). By allowing the body to burn fat during fasting periods, intermittent fasting directly targets liver fat and supports detoxification.

Furthermore, fasting activates a process called **autophagy**, during which the body cleans out damaged cells, including liver cells. Autophagy helps remove harmful substances from the liver, promoting repair and regeneration of healthy liver tissue. This detoxifying effect is beneficial in reversing fatty liver disease and improving overall liver health.

3. Weight Loss and Fatty Liver Disease Reversal

One of the most significant contributors to fatty liver disease is obesity. Excess body fat, particularly visceral fat, contributes to insulin resistance and liver inflammation. Intermittent fasting, by promoting weight loss, helps reduce the overall fat load on the body and liver. By encouraging gradual and sustainable fat loss, intermittent fasting reduces liver fat and improves the chances of reversing fatty liver disease.

Research has shown that even modest weight loss (5-10% of total body weight) can significantly improve liver health by reducing liver fat, inflammation, and fibrosis (scarring). Intermittent fasting provides a structured way to achieve this weight loss, making it an effective tool for people with fatty liver disease.

The Benefits of Intermittent Fasting for Fatty Liver Disease

Intermittent fasting offers a wide range of benefits specifically tailored to those dealing with fatty liver disease. These benefits include:

1. Improved Liver Enzyme Levels

Fatty liver disease often leads to elevated levels of liver enzymes (such as ALT and AST) in the blood. These enzymes are markers of liver inflammation and damage. Intermittent fasting has been shown to reduce the levels of these enzymes, indicating a reduction in liver inflammation and improvement in liver function.

2. Enhanced Fat Metabolism

Fasting enhances the liver's ability to process and burn fat. During fasting periods, insulin levels drop, and the body shifts to using fat as its primary source of energy. This promotes fat burning and helps to decrease fat accumulation in the liver, which is essential for reversing fatty liver disease.

3. Reduced Inflammation

Inflammation plays a major role in the progression of fatty liver disease, especially in the transition from NAFLD to NASH (non-alcoholic steatohepatitis), where liver inflammation and damage become more severe. Studies have shown that intermittent fasting can reduce markers of inflammation, which can help prevent further liver damage and slow the progression of fatty liver disease.

4. Improved Lipid Profile

Intermittent fasting has been found to improve cholesterol levels, including reducing LDL cholesterol (the "bad" cholesterol) and increasing HDL cholesterol (the "good" cholesterol). By improving lipid profiles, intermittent fasting helps to lower the risk of developing cardiovascular diseases, which are common in individuals with fatty liver disease.

5. Support for Liver Repair and Regeneration

Intermittent fasting triggers autophagy, a process where the body removes damaged cells and regenerates healthy ones. This process is particularly beneficial for the liver, as it can help repair liver tissue that has been damaged by fatty liver disease. The result is improved liver function and a reduced risk of liver fibrosis or cirrhosis.

How to Incorporate Intermittent Fasting for Fatty Liver Disease

If you're considering incorporating intermittent fasting into your routine to manage fatty liver disease, here are some tips to get started safely and effectively:

1. Consult Your Healthcare Provider

Before beginning any fasting regimen, especially if you have fatty liver disease or other health conditions, it's important to consult with your doctor or a registered dietitian. They can help determine whether intermittent fasting is appropriate for your health needs and provide personalized advice on how to proceed.

2. Start Slowly

If you're new to intermittent fasting, it's advisable to start slowly. Begin with a more gradual approach, such as the 12/12 method (12 hours of fasting and 12 hours of eating), and gradually increase the fasting window as your body adapts. For example, after a few weeks of 12-hour fasting, you might move to the 16/8 method, fasting for 16 hours and eating within an 8-hour window.

3. Focus on Nutrient-Dense, Liver-Healthy Foods

During your eating windows, prioritize foods that support liver health. This includes nutrient-dense vegetables, healthy fats (such as avocado, olive oil, and nuts), lean proteins, whole grains, and antioxidant-rich fruits. Avoid processed foods, sugars, and trans fats, as these can worsen liver damage and contribute to fat buildup.

4. Stay Hydrated

During fasting periods, it's important to stay hydrated. Drink plenty of water, herbal teas, or black coffee to help support liver detoxification and reduce hunger. Staying hydrated also helps maintain energy levels and supports your body's natural detox processes.

5. Listen to Your Body

Intermittent fasting can be an adjustment, especially in the beginning. Pay attention to your body's signals, and make sure to stop fasting if you experience severe hunger, dizziness, or weakness. Gradually increasing your fasting window and focusing on nutrient-rich meals can help ease the transition.

Chapter 4: 100+ Delicious Fatty Liver-Friendly Recipes for Every Meal of the Day

In this chapter, we will dive into a wide range of recipes that are not only delicious but also carefully crafted to support liver health. These recipes are designed to be rich in nutrients, antioxidants, and healthy fats that promote liver healing and detoxification. Whether you're just starting on your fatty liver-friendly journey or are looking for new ways to spice up your meals, this chapter will provide you with the tools you need to create meals that support your liver's health every day.

The Foundation of Liver-Healthy Recipes

When creating recipes for fatty liver disease, the goal is to include foods that are low in unhealthy fats, refined sugars, and processed ingredients, while focusing on nutrients that support liver function. Here's a breakdown of some essential principles for crafting liver-friendly meals:

- **Antioxidants**: Foods rich in antioxidants, such as leafy greens, berries, and colorful vegetables, help combat oxidative stress, a key contributor to liver damage.
- **Healthy Fats**: Incorporating healthy fats from sources like avocados, olive oil, and fatty fish can help reduce liver fat and support overall liver health.
- **Fiber**: High-fiber foods, such as whole grains, legumes, and vegetables, help regulate blood sugar and support digestion, reducing liver inflammation.
- **Lean Proteins**: Opting for lean protein sources, like chicken, turkey, tofu, and fish, helps reduce the intake of saturated fats and supports muscle health.

- **Herbs and Spices**: Many herbs and spices, including turmeric, garlic, and ginger, have liver-boosting properties that help reduce inflammation and improve detoxification.

Breakfast: Start Your Day with Liver-Supporting Nutrients

A healthy breakfast is essential to kickstart your metabolism and provide the necessary nutrients for a strong start to your day. These liver-healthy breakfast options are packed with fiber, antioxidants, and healthy fats to support liver function.

1. Avocado and Spinach Smoothie

Ingredients:

- 1 ripe avocado
- 1 cup spinach
- 1 small banana
- 1 tablespoon chia seeds
- 1 cup unsweetened almond milk
- A handful of ice cubes

Instructions:

1. Place all ingredients in a blender and blend until smooth.
2. Pour into a glass and enjoy!

Why it's good for the liver: This smoothie is packed with healthy fats from avocado and chia seeds, which help to reduce liver fat and inflammation. Spinach is rich in antioxidants and fiber, helping to support the detoxification process.

2. Oatmeal with Berries and Walnuts

Ingredients:

- 1/2 cup rolled oats
- 1 cup unsweetened almond milk
- 1/2 cup mixed berries (blueberries, strawberries, raspberries)
- 1 tablespoon ground flaxseeds
- 1 tablespoon walnuts, chopped

Instructions:

1. Cook the oats in almond milk according to package instructions.
2. Top with mixed berries, ground flaxseeds, and chopped walnuts.
3. Stir well and serve warm.

Why it's good for the liver: Oats are rich in fiber, which helps regulate blood sugar levels and reduce liver inflammation. Berries are loaded with antioxidants, and walnuts provide healthy fats that support liver health.

3. Turmeric Scrambled Eggs with Kale

Ingredients:

- 2 eggs
- 1 cup chopped kale

- 1/2 teaspoon turmeric powder
- 1/4 teaspoon black pepper
- 1 tablespoon olive oil
- Salt to taste

Instructions:

1. Heat olive oil in a skillet over medium heat.
2. Add the chopped kale and sauté for 2-3 minutes until wilted.
3. Crack the eggs into a bowl, add turmeric and black pepper, and whisk together.
4. Pour the eggs into the skillet and scramble with the kale until fully cooked.
5. Season with salt and serve warm.

Why it's good for the liver: Turmeric has powerful anti-inflammatory properties that can help reduce liver fat and inflammation. Kale is rich in antioxidants, and eggs provide a source of high-quality protein to support liver function.

Lunch: Nourishing and Filling Meals

Lunch should be a meal that keeps you satisfied and energized while providing essential nutrients for liver health. These lunch recipes are perfect for anyone with fatty liver disease, as they focus on liver-friendly ingredients like lean proteins, whole grains, and plenty of vegetables.

1. Grilled Salmon Salad with Olive Oil Dressing

Ingredients:

- 4 oz salmon fillet
- 2 cups mixed greens (arugula, spinach, kale)
- 1/4 cucumber, sliced
- 1/4 red onion, thinly sliced
- 1/2 avocado, sliced
- 1 tablespoon olive oil
- 1 tablespoon lemon juice
- Salt and pepper to taste

Instructions:

1. Grill the salmon until it reaches your desired level of doneness.
2. In a large bowl, combine the mixed greens, cucumber, onion, and avocado.
3. Flake the grilled salmon and add it to the salad.
4. Drizzle with olive oil and lemon juice, then toss gently to combine.
5. Season with salt and pepper to taste.

Why it's good for the liver: Salmon is a great source of omega-3 fatty acids, which help reduce inflammation and fat buildup in the liver. Olive oil provides healthy fats, and the vegetables add fiber and antioxidants to support liver detoxification.

2. Quinoa and Chickpea Bowl

Ingredients:

- 1/2 cup cooked quinoa
- 1/2 cup cooked chickpeas
- 1/4 cup diced cucumber

- 1/4 cup diced tomatoes
- 1 tablespoon olive oil
- 1 tablespoon lemon juice
- 1 teaspoon cumin
- Salt and pepper to taste

Instructions:

1. In a large bowl, combine the cooked quinoa and chickpeas.
2. Add the diced cucumber, tomatoes, olive oil, and lemon juice.
3. Sprinkle with cumin, salt, and pepper.
4. Toss gently and serve.

Why it's good for the liver: Quinoa and chickpeas are excellent plant-based sources of protein and fiber, helping to regulate blood sugar and reduce liver fat. The cumin and lemon juice add flavor while supporting digestion.

3. Grilled Chicken and Vegetable Stir-Fry

Ingredients:

- 4 oz boneless, skinless chicken breast, sliced
- 1 cup broccoli florets
- 1 bell pepper, sliced
- 1/2 onion, sliced
- 1 tablespoon olive oil
- 1 tablespoon low-sodium soy sauce
- 1 tablespoon sesame seeds

Instructions:

1. Heat olive oil in a skillet over medium-high heat.
2. Add the chicken slices and cook until browned and cooked through.
3. Add the vegetables and stir-fry for 4-5 minutes until tender-crisp.
4. Drizzle with soy sauce and sprinkle with sesame seeds.
5. Serve warm.

Why it's good for the liver: Chicken provides lean protein, while the vegetables provide fiber, vitamins, and antioxidants. Olive oil offers healthy fats, and sesame seeds add a crunchy, nutrient-dense topping.

Dinner: Light and Satisfying Evening Meals

Dinner should be a lighter meal that's easy to digest, providing a balance of nutrients that support liver repair and regeneration during sleep.

1. Baked Cod with Sweet Potato Mash

Ingredients:

- 4 oz cod fillet
- 1 medium sweet potato, peeled and cubed
- 1 tablespoon olive oil
- 1/2 teaspoon garlic powder
- 1/4 teaspoon paprika
- Salt and pepper to taste

Instructions:

1. Preheat your oven to 375°F (190°C).
2. Place the cod fillet on a baking sheet, drizzle with olive oil, and season with garlic powder, paprika, salt, and pepper.
3. Bake the cod for 15-20 minutes or until it flakes easily with a fork.
4. Meanwhile, boil the sweet potato cubes until tender (about 10-15 minutes), then mash them with a fork.
5. Serve the baked cod with the mashed sweet potatoes.

Why it's good for the liver: Cod is a lean protein with omega-3 fatty acids that help reduce liver inflammation, while sweet potatoes are rich in fiber and antioxidants, supporting liver detoxification.

2. Zucchini Noodles with Pesto and Grilled Shrimp

Ingredients:

- 2 medium zucchinis, spiralized into noodles
- 6 oz shrimp, peeled and deveined
- 1/4 cup pesto sauce (made with olive oil, basil, garlic, and nuts)
- 1 tablespoon olive oil
- Salt and pepper to taste

Instructions:

1. Heat olive oil in a skillet over medium heat.
2. Add the shrimp and cook for 2-3 minutes on each side until pink and cooked through.
3. In the same skillet, sauté the zucchini noodles for 2-3 minutes until just tender.

4. Toss the noodles with pesto sauce and top with grilled shrimp.
5. Serve warm.

Why it's good for the liver: Shrimp is a lean source of protein, and zucchini noodles are a low-carb, high-fiber alternative to pasta. Olive oil and pesto add healthy fats to the dish, while basil and garlic have liver-boosting properties.

Breakfast Recipes for Liver Health

A nutritious breakfast is the perfect way to kick-start your day, especially when you're focusing on improving liver health. Liver-boosting smoothies, overnight oats, and nutrient-dense egg dishes are ideal for providing your body with the right balance of essential nutrients. Packed with antioxidants, healthy fats, and fiber, these breakfast recipes are designed to nourish your liver and keep you feeling energized throughout the day.

Liver-Boosting Smoothies

Smoothies are a quick and convenient way to pack in liver-healthy nutrients. With a combination of fruits, vegetables, and superfoods, these smoothies are rich in antioxidants, vitamins, and healthy fats that support detoxification, reduce inflammation, and improve liver function.

1. Green Detox Smoothie

Ingredients:

- 1 cup spinach or kale
- 1/2 avocado
- 1/2 green apple
- 1/2 cucumber
- 1 tablespoon chia seeds
- 1 tablespoon lemon juice
- 1 cup unsweetened almond milk (or water)
- Ice cubes (optional)

Instructions:

1. Add all the ingredients to a blender.
2. Blend until smooth, adding more liquid as necessary.
3. Pour into a glass, and enjoy!

Why it's good for the liver:
Spinach and kale are rich in chlorophyll, which helps cleanse the liver and supports detoxification. Avocado provides healthy fats that support liver cell regeneration, while chia seeds offer omega-3 fatty acids to help reduce inflammation. Green apple and cucumber add a refreshing burst of antioxidants and hydration.

2. Berry Antioxidant Smoothie

Ingredients:

- 1/2 cup blueberries (fresh or frozen)
- 1/2 cup strawberries (fresh or frozen)
- 1 tablespoon ground flaxseeds
- 1/2 cup Greek yogurt (unsweetened)
- 1 tablespoon honey (optional)
- 1 cup unsweetened almond milk

Instructions:

1. Place all the ingredients in a blender.
2. Blend until creamy and smooth.
3. Serve immediately and enjoy!

Why it's good for the liver:
Berries, particularly blueberries and strawberries, are rich in antioxidants that combat oxidative stress in the liver. Flaxseeds provide fiber and healthy omega-3 fatty acids, promoting digestion and reducing inflammation. Greek yogurt adds a source of probiotics, which support gut health—a vital aspect of overall liver health.

3. Tropical Liver Detox Smoothie

Ingredients:

- 1/2 cup pineapple (fresh or frozen)
- 1/2 cup mango (fresh or frozen)
- 1 tablespoon coconut oil
- 1/4 teaspoon turmeric powder
- 1 cup coconut water
- 1 tablespoon chia seeds
- 1/2 lime, juiced

Instructions:

1. Combine all ingredients in a blender.
2. Blend until smooth and creamy.
3. Pour into a glass and serve chilled.

Why it's good for the liver:
Pineapple and mango are both rich in vitamin C, which aids in detoxification, and bromelain (found in pineapple) helps reduce inflammation. Coconut oil provides healthy fats, while turmeric's active compound, curcumin, has potent anti-inflammatory and liver-protective properties. Chia seeds offer fiber and omega-3 fatty acids, which support liver function.

Overnight Oats for Liver Health

Overnight oats are a simple, no-cook option that can be prepared the night before and enjoyed the next morning. They are fiber-rich, provide steady energy throughout the morning, and are perfect for supporting liver health with their high antioxidant content and healthy fats.

1. Antioxidant-Packed Chia Pudding

Ingredients:

- 1/2 cup rolled oats
- 1 tablespoon chia seeds
- 1/2 cup unsweetened almond milk
- 1/4 cup blueberries
- 1/4 cup chopped walnuts
- 1 teaspoon honey (optional)

Instructions:

1. In a jar or container, combine oats, chia seeds, and almond milk.
2. Stir well and cover.

3. Let it sit in the fridge overnight.
4. The next morning, top with blueberries, walnuts, and honey.
5. Enjoy!

Why it's good for the liver:
Chia seeds are packed with fiber, omega-3 fatty acids, and antioxidants, making them a powerful addition to your liver-friendly breakfast. Blueberries provide antioxidants that help reduce oxidative stress, while walnuts contain healthy fats and vitamin E that support liver function.

2. Cinnamon Apple Overnight Oats

Ingredients:

- 1/2 cup rolled oats
- 1 tablespoon flaxseeds
- 1/2 cup unsweetened almond milk
- 1/2 apple, diced
- 1/4 teaspoon cinnamon
- 1 tablespoon walnuts, chopped
- 1 teaspoon honey (optional)

Instructions:

1. In a jar or container, combine oats, flaxseeds, and almond milk.
2. Stir well and cover.
3. Refrigerate overnight.
4. The next morning, top with diced apple, cinnamon, walnuts, and honey.
5. Enjoy!

Why it's good for the liver:
Flaxseeds and walnuts provide healthy omega-3s and fiber, which help reduce inflammation and promote liver detoxification. Apples are a great source of fiber and antioxidants, while cinnamon has anti-inflammatory properties that can support liver health.

3. Chocolate-Almond Overnight Oats

Ingredients:

- 1/2 cup rolled oats
- 1 tablespoon almond butter
- 1 tablespoon raw cacao powder
- 1/2 cup unsweetened almond milk
- 1 teaspoon chia seeds
- 1 tablespoon sliced almonds

Instructions:

1. In a jar or container, combine oats, almond butter, cacao powder, almond milk, and chia seeds.
2. Stir until well combined, then cover and refrigerate overnight.
3. In the morning, top with sliced almonds and enjoy!

Why it's good for the liver:
Cacao is rich in flavonoids, which have been shown to reduce liver inflammation and promote detoxification. Almond butter and sliced almonds provide healthy fats, which support liver repair, while chia seeds offer fiber and omega-3 fatty acids.

Nutrient-Dense Egg Dishes for Liver Health

Eggs are an excellent source of high-quality protein and essential nutrients, including vitamin B12 and choline, which support liver function. In this section, we'll focus on easy-to-make, liver-friendly egg dishes that can be enjoyed for breakfast.

1. Spinach and Mushroom Scrambled Eggs

Ingredients:

- 2 eggs
- 1/2 cup fresh spinach, chopped
- 1/2 cup mushrooms, sliced
- 1 tablespoon olive oil
- 1/4 teaspoon turmeric powder
- Salt and pepper to taste

Instructions:

1. Heat olive oil in a skillet over medium heat.
2. Add mushrooms and sauté for 2-3 minutes until tender.
3. Add spinach and cook until wilted, about 1-2 minutes.
4. Crack eggs into the skillet, sprinkle with turmeric, salt, and pepper, and scramble until fully cooked.
5. Serve immediately.

Why it's good for the liver:
Spinach and mushrooms are rich in antioxidants and fiber, which help protect the liver from oxidative damage. The turmeric in this dish has anti-inflammatory properties that

support liver detoxification. Eggs provide high-quality protein and choline, which is essential for liver function and fat metabolism.

2. Avocado and Tomato Egg Bowl

Ingredients:

- 2 eggs
- 1/2 avocado, sliced
- 1/2 tomato, diced
- 1 tablespoon olive oil
- Salt and pepper to taste
- Fresh cilantro (optional)

Instructions:

1. Heat olive oil in a skillet over medium heat.
2. Crack eggs into the skillet and cook them to your desired doneness (sunny-side up, scrambled, etc.).
3. Arrange eggs on a plate and top with avocado, diced tomato, and fresh cilantro.
4. Season with salt and pepper to taste.

Why it's good for the liver:
Avocados are loaded with healthy fats that help reduce liver fat and support liver regeneration. Tomatoes provide antioxidants like lycopene, which helps protect the liver from damage. Eggs provide protein and choline, vital for liver function.

3. Egg and Veggie Breakfast Muffins

Ingredients:

- 4 eggs
- 1/2 cup bell peppers, chopped
- 1/4 cup onion, chopped
- 1/4 cup spinach, chopped
- 1/4 teaspoon garlic powder
- 1/4 teaspoon black pepper
- Salt to taste

Instructions:

1. Preheat your oven to 350°F (175°C).
2. Whisk eggs in a bowl, then stir in the chopped vegetables, garlic powder, black pepper, and salt.
3. Pour the mixture into a muffin tin, filling each cup about 3/4 full.
4. Bake for 15-18 minutes, or until the eggs are set.
5. Let cool slightly and enjoy!

Why it's good for the liver:
This recipe is full of nutrient-dense vegetables that provide fiber, vitamins, and antioxidants. Eggs supply high-quality protein and choline, supporting liver health. The combination of ingredients supports detoxification, helps reduce inflammation, and promotes overall liver function.

Lunch Recipes for Liver Health

Lunchtime offers a great opportunity to refuel your body with nutrient-packed, liver-friendly meals. High-fiber salads, lean protein bowls, and easy-to-make wraps can be both delicious and effective in promoting liver health. By including antioxidant-rich vegetables, healthy fats, and lean proteins, these lunch recipes support liver detoxification, improve liver function, and keep you energized for the rest of the day.

High-Fiber Salads

Salads are a wonderful way to incorporate a variety of liver-healthy foods, particularly vegetables that are high in fiber and antioxidants. Fiber helps with digestion and liver detoxification, while the added vegetables provide essential vitamins and minerals that support liver health.

1. Kale and Quinoa Detox Salad

Ingredients:

- 2 cups kale, chopped
- 1/2 cup cooked quinoa
- 1/4 cup cherry tomatoes, halved
- 1/4 cup cucumber, diced
- 1 tablespoon olive oil
- 1 tablespoon lemon juice
- 1 tablespoon apple cider vinegar
- 1 tablespoon chia seeds
- Salt and pepper to taste

Instructions:

1. In a large bowl, combine the kale, quinoa, cherry tomatoes, and cucumber.
2. In a small bowl, whisk together the olive oil, lemon juice, apple cider vinegar, chia seeds, salt, and pepper.
3. Pour the dressing over the salad and toss well.

4. Serve immediately or refrigerate for later.

Why it's good for the liver:
Kale is a powerhouse vegetable rich in antioxidants and fiber, both of which support liver detoxification and reduce oxidative stress. Quinoa adds a plant-based source of protein and fiber. Chia seeds provide omega-3 fatty acids, which help reduce liver inflammation. Lemon juice and apple cider vinegar help alkalize the body and support liver function.

2. Mediterranean Chickpea Salad

Ingredients:

- 1 cup cooked chickpeas
- 1/2 cup cucumber, diced
- 1/4 cup red onion, thinly sliced
- 1/4 cup Kalamata olives, chopped
- 1/4 cup feta cheese, crumbled (optional)
- 1 tablespoon olive oil
- 1 tablespoon red wine vinegar
- 1 teaspoon dried oregano
- Salt and pepper to taste

Instructions:

1. In a large bowl, combine the chickpeas, cucumber, red onion, olives, and feta cheese (if using).
2. In a small bowl, whisk together the olive oil, red wine vinegar, oregano, salt, and pepper.
3. Pour the dressing over the salad and toss gently.
4. Serve immediately or store in the fridge for up to a day.

Why it's good for the liver:
Chickpeas are an excellent source of fiber and plant-based protein, which support liver function and help maintain a healthy weight. Cucumber and red onion offer anti-inflammatory compounds and antioxidants that help reduce liver stress. Olive oil is rich in healthy fats, which promote liver regeneration. The Mediterranean ingredients are all nutrient-dense and promote overall liver health.

3. Sweet Potato and Black Bean Salad

Ingredients:

- 1 medium sweet potato, roasted and cubed
- 1/2 cup cooked black beans
- 1/4 cup red bell pepper, diced
- 1/4 cup green onions, chopped
- 1 tablespoon olive oil
- 1 tablespoon lime juice
- 1 teaspoon cumin
- 1 tablespoon cilantro, chopped
- Salt and pepper to taste

Instructions:

1. Preheat the oven to 400°F (200°C). Roast the sweet potato cubes on a baking sheet with a drizzle of olive oil and a pinch of salt for 25-30 minutes, or until tender.
2. In a large bowl, combine the roasted sweet potato, black beans, red bell pepper, and green onions.
3. In a small bowl, whisk together olive oil, lime juice, cumin, cilantro, salt, and pepper.
4. Pour the dressing over the salad and toss gently.

5. Serve warm or chilled.

Why it's good for the liver:
Sweet potatoes are rich in beta-carotene and fiber, which help support liver function and detoxification. Black beans provide plant-based protein and fiber, which are crucial for weight management and liver health. Lime juice and cilantro add a burst of antioxidants that support liver cleansing. This salad is nutrient-dense, filling, and anti-inflammatory, making it ideal for liver health.

Lean Protein Bowls

Protein is essential for liver repair and detoxification. When paired with fiber-rich vegetables and healthy fats, lean proteins can help you maintain a balanced, liver-healthy diet. These bowls are not only tasty but also provide your liver with the nutrients it needs to thrive.

1. Grilled Salmon and Veggie Bowl

Ingredients:

- 1 salmon fillet (about 6 oz)
- 1/2 cup cooked quinoa
- 1/2 cup steamed broccoli
- 1/2 cup roasted sweet potatoes, cubed
- 1 tablespoon olive oil
- 1 tablespoon lemon juice
- Salt and pepper to taste

Instructions:

1. Preheat the grill or a grill pan over medium-high heat. Season the salmon with olive oil, salt, and pepper.
2. Grill the salmon for 3-4 minutes per side, or until it is fully cooked.
3. Assemble the bowl with quinoa, steamed broccoli, roasted sweet potatoes, and grilled salmon.
4. Drizzle with lemon juice and serve immediately.

Why it's good for the liver:
Salmon is rich in omega-3 fatty acids, which help reduce inflammation and support liver regeneration. Quinoa provides fiber and protein, while sweet potatoes are packed with antioxidants. Broccoli contains sulforaphane, a compound that helps activate liver detoxification enzymes. This bowl is a complete, nutrient-dense meal that nourishes the liver and supports overall health.

2. Chicken and Avocado Power Bowl

Ingredients:

- 1 chicken breast (grilled or baked)
- 1/2 avocado, sliced
- 1/2 cup brown rice
- 1/2 cup spinach, sautéed
- 1 tablespoon olive oil
- 1 tablespoon balsamic vinegar
- Salt and pepper to taste

Instructions:

1. Grill or bake the chicken breast until fully cooked. Slice it into thin strips.

2. Cook brown rice according to package instructions.
3. In a skillet, sauté the spinach with a little olive oil until wilted.
4. Assemble the bowl with brown rice, sautéed spinach, avocado slices, and chicken.
5. Drizzle with balsamic vinegar, season with salt and pepper, and serve.

Why it's good for the liver:
Chicken is a lean source of protein that supports liver repair and detoxification. Avocado provides healthy monounsaturated fats that help reduce liver fat. Brown rice adds fiber and helps regulate blood sugar levels. Spinach offers antioxidants and anti-inflammatory compounds that support liver function. This bowl is a perfect combination of healthy fats, protein, and fiber to nourish the liver.

3. Tofu and Veggie Stir-Fry Bowl

Ingredients:

- 1/2 block firm tofu, cubed
- 1 cup mixed bell peppers, sliced
- 1/2 cup snap peas
- 1/4 cup carrots, julienned
- 2 tablespoons tamari (or soy sauce)
- 1 tablespoon sesame oil
- 1 tablespoon rice vinegar
- 1 tablespoon sesame seeds
- 1/2 teaspoon ginger, grated

Instructions:

1. Press tofu to remove excess water, then cut into cubes.
2. Heat sesame oil in a skillet over medium heat. Add tofu and cook until golden and crispy, about 7-8 minutes.
3. Remove tofu and set aside. In the same skillet, sauté the bell peppers, snap peas, and carrots for 3-4 minutes, or until tender-crisp.
4. Add the tofu back to the skillet along with tamari, rice vinegar, and grated ginger. Stir to coat.
5. Serve the stir-fry in a bowl, topped with sesame seeds.

Why it's good for the liver:
Tofu is a great source of plant-based protein and contains antioxidants that support liver health. Bell peppers are rich in vitamin C and antioxidants, while snap peas and carrots add fiber and essential nutrients. Sesame oil and seeds offer healthy fats that promote liver regeneration and reduce inflammation. This stir-fry bowl is a delicious, liver-friendly option for lunch.

Easy-to-Make Wraps

Wraps are a convenient, on-the-go option for lunch, packed with protein, fiber, and liver-boosting nutrients. By filling your wrap with antioxidant-rich veggies, lean proteins, and healthy fats, you can create a quick meal that supports your liver.

1. Turkey and Avocado Lettuce Wraps

Ingredients:

- 4 large lettuce leaves (e.g., Romaine or Butterhead)
- 4 oz lean turkey breast, sliced

- 1/2 avocado, sliced
- 1/4 cup shredded carrots
- 1 tablespoon mustard or hummus
- Salt and pepper to taste

Instructions:

1. Lay out the lettuce leaves and spread a thin layer of mustard or hummus on each.
2. Place turkey slices, avocado, and shredded carrots in the center of each lettuce leaf.
3. Season with salt and pepper, then wrap and serve immediately.

Why it's good for the liver:
Turkey is a lean source of protein that supports liver regeneration. Avocado provides healthy fats that reduce liver fat accumulation, while carrots offer beta-carotene and fiber. Mustard or hummus adds flavor without excessive calories or unhealthy fats. These wraps are light, filling, and perfect for supporting liver health.

2. Veggie and Hummus Wrap

Ingredients:

- 1 whole-grain wrap or tortilla
- 1/4 cup hummus
- 1/2 cup mixed greens
- 1/4 cup cucumber, sliced
- 1/4 cup red bell pepper, sliced
- 1/4 cup shredded red cabbage

Instructions:

1. Lay the wrap flat and spread hummus evenly across the surface.
2. Layer the mixed greens, cucumber, red bell pepper, and red cabbage on top.
3. Roll up the wrap, slice in half, and serve.

Why it's good for the liver:
Hummus is a great source of healthy fats, fiber, and plant-based protein. The mixed greens, cucumber, and red cabbage provide antioxidant-rich vegetables that help detoxify the liver. The whole-grain wrap ensures you get a good amount of fiber to promote liver health and digestion. This wrap is a light, satisfying option for a quick and nutritious lunch.

Dinner Recipes for Liver Health

Dinner is the perfect time to enjoy a balanced, liver-friendly meal that nourishes the body and helps support its detoxification and repair processes overnight. A dinner rich in low-fat, anti-inflammatory ingredients—such as healthy fats, lean proteins, and liver-friendly vegetables—can promote liver function, reduce oxidative stress, and improve overall health. Here are some delicious, nutrient-dense dinner recipes that support liver health.

1. Grilled Lemon Herb Chicken with Roasted Vegetables

Ingredients:

- 2 boneless, skinless chicken breasts
- 1 tablespoon olive oil
- 1 tablespoon lemon juice
- 1 teaspoon dried oregano
- 1/2 teaspoon garlic powder
- Salt and pepper to taste
- 1 cup Brussels sprouts, halved
- 1 small sweet potato, diced
- 1 tablespoon olive oil
- 1 teaspoon rosemary, chopped
- 1/2 teaspoon turmeric
- 1/2 teaspoon black pepper

Instructions:

1. Preheat the grill or a grill pan over medium heat.
2. In a small bowl, mix olive oil, lemon juice, oregano, garlic powder, salt, and pepper. Coat the chicken breasts with the marinade and set aside for at least 15 minutes.
3. While the chicken marinates, preheat the oven to 400°F (200°C).
4. Toss Brussels sprouts and sweet potato with olive oil, rosemary, turmeric, black pepper, salt, and pepper. Spread the vegetables in a single layer on a baking sheet and roast for 25-30 minutes, turning halfway through, until tender and golden.
5. Grill the chicken for 5-7 minutes per side or until fully cooked.
6. Serve the grilled chicken with roasted vegetables on the side.

Why it's good for the liver:
Chicken is a lean protein that helps support liver repair. Olive oil is rich in healthy monounsaturated fats, which reduce inflammation and promote liver function. Brussels sprouts are part of the cruciferous vegetable family, which contains compounds that support liver detoxification. Sweet potatoes are high in beta-carotene and fiber, both of which are beneficial for liver health. The combination of herbs and spices like turmeric adds powerful anti-inflammatory properties to the meal.

2. Baked Salmon with Avocado Salsa

Ingredients:

- 2 salmon fillets (6 oz each)
- 1 tablespoon olive oil
- 1 teaspoon garlic powder
- 1 teaspoon smoked paprika
- Salt and pepper to taste
- 1 avocado, diced
- 1/4 cup red onion, finely chopped
- 1/2 cup cherry tomatoes, halved
- 1 tablespoon lime juice
- 1 tablespoon cilantro, chopped

Instructions:

1. Preheat the oven to 375°F (190°C).
2. Rub the salmon fillets with olive oil, garlic powder, smoked paprika, salt, and pepper.

3. Place the fillets on a baking sheet lined with parchment paper and bake for 12-15 minutes, or until the salmon flakes easily with a fork.
4. While the salmon is baking, prepare the avocado salsa by combining diced avocado, red onion, cherry tomatoes, lime juice, and cilantro in a small bowl. Stir gently to combine.
5. Once the salmon is ready, top each fillet with a generous scoop of avocado salsa and serve immediately.

Why it's good for the liver:
Salmon is rich in omega-3 fatty acids, which have been shown to reduce liver fat and inflammation. The healthy fats from avocado provide additional anti-inflammatory benefits and support liver cell regeneration. Lime juice is a natural detoxifier that supports liver function. This dish is rich in antioxidants, healthy fats, and lean protein, making it an excellent choice for liver health.

3. Spaghetti Squash Primavera

Ingredients:

- 1 medium spaghetti squash
- 1 tablespoon olive oil
- 1 small zucchini, thinly sliced
- 1 bell pepper, thinly sliced
- 1/2 cup cherry tomatoes, halved
- 1/4 cup red onion, thinly sliced
- 1 teaspoon garlic powder
- Salt and pepper to taste
- Fresh basil, chopped for garnish

- 2 tablespoons nutritional yeast (optional)

Instructions:

1. Preheat the oven to 400°F (200°C).
2. Cut the spaghetti squash in half lengthwise and scoop out the seeds. Drizzle the flesh with olive oil, sprinkle with salt and pepper, and place the squash halves cut-side down on a baking sheet. Roast for 30-40 minutes or until the squash is tender and easily shredded with a fork.
3. While the squash is roasting, heat olive oil in a large skillet over medium heat. Add zucchini, bell pepper, cherry tomatoes, and red onion. Sauté for 5-7 minutes, or until the vegetables are tender.
4. Once the squash is ready, use a fork to shred the flesh into spaghetti-like strands.
5. Add the sautéed vegetables to the shredded squash and toss to combine. Season with garlic powder, salt, and pepper.
6. Garnish with fresh basil and nutritional yeast if desired, and serve.

Why it's good for the liver:
Spaghetti squash is a low-carb, high-fiber vegetable that supports digestion and liver health. The colorful array of vegetables in this dish provides antioxidants and anti-inflammatory compounds that support detoxification and reduce liver stress. Olive oil adds healthy fats to the meal, promoting liver cell repair. This dish is light, filling, and ideal for promoting liver health.

4. Stir-Fried Tofu with Vegetables

Ingredients:

- 1 block firm tofu, pressed and cubed
- 1 tablespoon sesame oil
- 1 cup broccoli florets
- 1/2 cup red bell pepper, sliced
- 1/2 cup snap peas
- 1/4 cup carrots, julienned
- 2 tablespoons tamari or soy sauce (low-sodium)
- 1 tablespoon rice vinegar
- 1 teaspoon ginger, freshly grated
- 1 teaspoon garlic, minced
- 1 tablespoon sesame seeds (optional)
- Fresh cilantro, chopped for garnish

Instructions:

1. Press the tofu to remove excess water, then cut it into cubes.
2. Heat sesame oil in a large skillet or wok over medium heat. Add tofu cubes and cook until golden brown and crispy on all sides, about 8 minutes.
3. Add the broccoli, bell pepper, snap peas, and carrots to the skillet and stir-fry for another 5-7 minutes, or until the vegetables are tender-crisp.
4. In a small bowl, mix tamari or soy sauce, rice vinegar, ginger, and garlic. Pour the sauce over the tofu and vegetables and stir well to coat.
5. Garnish with sesame seeds and fresh cilantro, and serve immediately.

Why it's good for the liver:
Tofu is a great plant-based protein that supports liver repair and regeneration. The combination of sesame oil and sesame seeds provides healthy fats that reduce liver inflammation. The vegetables are full of vitamins, antioxidants, and fiber, which help detoxify the liver and support overall health. Ginger and garlic are both known for their anti-inflammatory properties and contribute to better liver function.

5. Lentil and Vegetable Curry

Ingredients:

- 1 cup dried lentils, rinsed
- 1 tablespoon coconut oil
- 1 onion, chopped
- 2 cloves garlic, minced
- 1 tablespoon ginger, grated
- 1 teaspoon turmeric
- 1 teaspoon cumin
- 1 teaspoon coriander
- 1 can (14 oz) diced tomatoes
- 1 cup spinach, chopped
- 1 cup coconut milk (light)
- Salt and pepper to taste
- Fresh cilantro for garnish

Instructions:

1. In a large pot, heat coconut oil over medium heat. Add onion, garlic, and ginger, and sauté until fragrant, about 5 minutes.

2. Stir in the turmeric, cumin, and coriander, and cook for 1-2 minutes to release the flavors.
3. Add the lentils, diced tomatoes, coconut milk, and 2 cups of water to the pot. Bring to a boil, then reduce to a simmer and cook for 25-30 minutes, or until the lentils are tender.
4. Stir in the spinach and cook for another 5 minutes, or until wilted.
5. Season with salt and pepper to taste, and garnish with fresh cilantro before serving.

Why it's good for the liver:
Lentils are a great source of plant-based protein and fiber, which support liver detoxification and digestion. Turmeric and ginger are potent anti-inflammatory spices that help reduce liver inflammation. Coconut milk provides healthy fats that help absorb fat-soluble nutrients. This curry is a hearty, warming dish that's both delicious and supportive of liver health.

Snacks and Desserts for Liver Health

Snacks and desserts can be a great way to satisfy cravings while nourishing your liver and balancing blood sugar levels. The key to liver-friendly treats is to incorporate ingredients that reduce inflammation, support detoxification, and help maintain steady blood sugar levels. By focusing on whole, unprocessed foods that are low in sugar and high in fiber, healthy fats, and antioxidants, you can indulge in sweet bites that promote liver health without compromising your wellness goals.

1. Chia Seed Pudding with Berries

Ingredients:

- 1/4 cup chia seeds
- 1 cup unsweetened almond milk (or any plant-based milk)
- 1 teaspoon vanilla extract
- 1/2 teaspoon ground cinnamon
- 1 tablespoon maple syrup or honey (optional, for sweetness)
- 1/2 cup mixed berries (blueberries, raspberries, strawberries)
- 1 tablespoon chopped almonds (optional, for crunch)

Instructions:

1. In a mixing bowl, combine chia seeds, almond milk, vanilla extract, cinnamon, and sweetener (if using).
2. Stir well and let the mixture sit for about 10 minutes. Then, stir again to prevent clumping.
3. Cover the bowl and refrigerate for at least 2 hours or overnight to allow the chia seeds to expand and thicken into a pudding-like consistency.
4. Before serving, top with fresh mixed berries and chopped almonds for added texture and nutrients.
5. Serve chilled.

Why it's good for the liver:
Chia seeds are rich in fiber, omega-3 fatty acids, and antioxidants, all of which support liver health by reducing inflammation and helping the liver detoxify. The berries

provide additional antioxidants like anthocyanins, which protect liver cells from oxidative damage. Cinnamon helps regulate blood sugar levels, making this treat perfect for those managing insulin resistance or fatty liver disease.

2. Avocado Chocolate Mousse

Ingredients:

- 1 ripe avocado
- 2 tablespoons unsweetened cocoa powder
- 2 tablespoons maple syrup or honey (adjust to taste)
- 1 teaspoon vanilla extract
- Pinch of sea salt
- 1/4 cup unsweetened almond milk (or any plant-based milk)
- Dark chocolate shavings (optional, for garnish)

Instructions:

1. In a blender or food processor, combine the avocado, cocoa powder, maple syrup, vanilla extract, sea salt, and almond milk.
2. Blend until smooth and creamy, scraping down the sides if necessary.
3. Taste and adjust sweetness if needed by adding a little more maple syrup or honey.
4. Spoon the mousse into small serving cups and refrigerate for at least 30 minutes to allow the flavors to meld together.
5. Before serving, garnish with dark chocolate shavings or a sprinkle of cacao nibs.

Why it's good for the liver:
Avocado is rich in healthy monounsaturated fats, which support liver health by reducing inflammation and promoting detoxification. The cocoa powder is full of antioxidants, particularly flavonoids, that help protect liver cells. This dessert is naturally sweetened with maple syrup or honey, which are both better alternatives to refined sugars that can disrupt liver function and blood sugar balance.

3. Roasted Almonds with Turmeric and Cinnamon

Ingredients:

- 1 cup raw almonds
- 1 tablespoon olive oil or coconut oil
- 1 teaspoon ground turmeric
- 1/2 teaspoon ground cinnamon
- 1/4 teaspoon black pepper
- Pinch of sea salt
- 1 teaspoon honey (optional)

Instructions:

1. Preheat the oven to 350°F (175°C).
2. In a bowl, toss the almonds with olive oil, turmeric, cinnamon, black pepper, and salt.
3. Spread the almonds evenly on a baking sheet in a single layer.
4. Roast for 15-20 minutes, stirring halfway through, until golden brown and fragrant.

5. Remove from the oven and allow the almonds to cool. If you like a touch of sweetness, drizzle the almonds with honey while they're still warm.
6. Serve as a crunchy snack or store in an airtight container.

Why it's good for the liver:
Almonds are rich in healthy fats, protein, and fiber, making them an excellent snack for maintaining blood sugar levels. Turmeric, with its active compound curcumin, is a potent anti-inflammatory that supports liver detoxification. Cinnamon helps stabilize blood sugar, while black pepper enhances the bioavailability of curcumin, making this snack even more effective in supporting liver health.

4. Apple Slices with Almond Butter and Cinnamon

Ingredients:

- 1 medium apple (such as Granny Smith or Fuji), sliced
- 2 tablespoons almond butter (or any nut butter of choice)
- 1/4 teaspoon ground cinnamon
- 1 teaspoon chia seeds (optional, for added fiber and omega-3s)

Instructions:

1. Slice the apple into thin wedges and arrange them on a plate.
2. Drizzle the almond butter over the apple slices or serve it on the side for dipping.

3. Sprinkle the apple slices with cinnamon and chia seeds, if using.
4. Enjoy immediately.

Why it's good for the liver:
Apples are rich in fiber, particularly pectin, which helps support digestion and liver detoxification. Almond butter provides healthy fats and protein, both of which help balance blood sugar levels and support liver cell regeneration. Cinnamon adds a sweet and aromatic touch, while also stabilizing blood sugar, making this a perfect snack for liver health.

5. Coconut Yogurt Parfait with Granola and Fresh Fruit

Ingredients:

- 1 cup unsweetened coconut yogurt (or any plant-based yogurt)
- 1/4 cup homemade or store-bought granola (preferably low-sugar)
- 1/2 cup mixed fresh fruit (e.g., berries, kiwi, mango, or pomegranate seeds)
- 1 tablespoon chia seeds
- 1 teaspoon honey or maple syrup (optional)

Instructions:

1. In a bowl or jar, layer coconut yogurt, granola, and fresh fruit.

2. Sprinkle chia seeds on top and drizzle with honey or maple syrup if desired.
3. Repeat the layers as desired and enjoy immediately or refrigerate for later.

Why it's good for the liver:
Coconut yogurt is a dairy-free alternative that contains probiotics to support gut health, which is essential for overall detoxification. The granola provides fiber, while fresh fruit is rich in antioxidants, vitamins, and minerals that protect the liver from oxidative stress. Chia seeds add healthy omega-3 fatty acids and fiber, promoting liver detoxification and balancing blood sugar levels.

6. Baked Cinnamon Apples with Walnuts

Ingredients:

- 2 medium apples, cored
- 1/4 cup walnuts, chopped
- 1 tablespoon raisins or dried cranberries
- 1/2 teaspoon cinnamon
- 1/2 teaspoon ground ginger
- 1 tablespoon maple syrup or honey (optional)
- 1/2 cup water

Instructions:

1. Preheat the oven to 350°F (175°C).
2. Core the apples and place them in a baking dish.

3. In a small bowl, combine the chopped walnuts, raisins or cranberries, cinnamon, ginger, and maple syrup (if using).
4. Stuff the apples with the mixture and place them in the baking dish.
5. Pour water into the bottom of the baking dish to help steam the apples.
6. Cover with foil and bake for 25-30 minutes or until the apples are tender.
7. Serve warm, topped with additional walnuts or a drizzle of honey.

Why it's good for the liver:
Apples, like in the previous recipe, provide fiber and antioxidants that support liver health. Walnuts are rich in omega-3 fatty acids and antioxidants that help reduce liver inflammation. Cinnamon and ginger are anti-inflammatory spices that help promote blood sugar balance, which is crucial for those managing fatty liver disease.

Special Recipe Feature: Gluten-Free, Dairy-Free, and Other Modifications for Specific Dietary Needs

When following a liver-friendly diet, it's essential to be mindful of not only the ingredients that promote liver health but also any additional dietary restrictions or preferences. Many people have specific needs such as gluten intolerance, dairy sensitivities, or other food allergies that must be taken into account. The good news is that a fatty liver diet can be easily tailored to accommodate these needs without sacrificing taste or nutritional value. In this section, we'll explore how to modify liver-healthy recipes to be gluten-free, dairy-free, and suited for other dietary preferences, ensuring that everyone can benefit from a liver-friendly lifestyle.

1. Gluten-Free Modifications

Gluten is a protein found in wheat, barley, and rye, and for those with celiac disease or gluten sensitivity, it can cause inflammation, digestive distress, and contribute to various autoimmune reactions. A gluten-free diet can be beneficial for individuals who need to reduce inflammation and support overall liver function. Fortunately, there are plenty of naturally gluten-free ingredients that are both delicious and liver-friendly.

How to modify recipes:

- **Flour Alternatives**: Substitute traditional wheat flour with gluten-free flours such as almond flour, coconut flour, rice flour, or chickpea flour. These flours provide healthy fats and fiber, which are beneficial for liver health. For example, gluten-free almond flour is a great choice for making low-carb, liver-supportive baked goods.
- **Oats**: Choose certified gluten-free oats for recipes like overnight oats or oatmeal. Many oats are processed in facilities that also handle wheat, so it's important to look for the "gluten-free" label to ensure safety for those with sensitivities.
- **Pasta**: For pasta dishes, try using gluten-free pasta made from quinoa, brown rice, or chickpea flour. These alternatives are not only gluten-free but also high in fiber and protein.

- **Bread**: Replace regular bread with gluten-free bread or homemade gluten-free bread made from almond or coconut flour. Gluten-free wraps can be used for wraps and sandwiches, providing a satisfying and liver-healthy meal option.

Example Recipe Modification:

- **Gluten-Free Avocado Toast**
  Swap out regular whole-grain bread for gluten-free bread or rice cakes. Top with mashed avocado, a drizzle of olive oil, and a sprinkle of chia seeds and chili flakes for added fiber and healthy fats.

2. Dairy-Free Modifications

Dairy products, such as milk, cheese, and butter, can cause inflammation and digestive discomfort in some individuals, particularly those with lactose intolerance or dairy sensitivities. Many dairy products are also high in saturated fats, which may not be ideal for those looking to support liver health. Adopting dairy-free alternatives is a great way to create a more anti-inflammatory, liver-friendly meal plan.

How to modify recipes:

- **Milk Substitutes**: Use plant-based milks such as almond milk, coconut milk, oat milk, or cashew milk as alternatives to cow's milk. These milk substitutes are naturally low in calories and free from saturated fat, making them great for liver health.

- **Cheese Substitutes**: There are a variety of plant-based cheese alternatives available, made from nuts (like cashews) or coconut milk, that can replace traditional cheese in recipes. Vegan cheeses are often lower in fat and can be used in salads, wraps, or baked dishes.
- **Butter Substitutes**: Replace butter with plant-based oils such as olive oil, avocado oil, or coconut oil. These oils contain healthy fats that support liver function and help reduce inflammation.
- **Yogurt Alternatives**: Swap regular dairy yogurt for coconut milk yogurt, almond milk yogurt, or soy yogurt. These alternatives often contain probiotics that support gut health, which is crucial for overall detoxification.

Example Recipe Modification:

- **Dairy-Free Smoothie Bowl**
  Blend unsweetened almond milk with frozen berries, spinach, and a scoop of plant-based protein powder. Top with gluten-free granola, chia seeds, and a drizzle of almond butter. This smoothie bowl is packed with fiber, antioxidants, and healthy fats, all of which are great for liver health.

3. Nut-Free and Seed-Free Modifications

For those with nut or seed allergies, many liver-healthy recipes can still be adapted to avoid nuts and seeds without compromising on taste or nutrition. Both nuts and seeds are excellent sources of healthy fats, fiber, and antioxidants, but there are plenty of other options that can provide similar benefits.

How to modify recipes:

- **Healthy Fats**: If a recipe calls for nuts, replace them with other healthy fat sources such as avocado, olives, or coconut. Avocados are rich in monounsaturated fats, which help reduce liver inflammation, while olives provide a dose of antioxidants.
- **Fiber**: If a recipe calls for chia seeds, flaxseeds, or sunflower seeds, you can substitute these with oats, psyllium husk, or hemp seeds (if tolerated). These are all fiber-rich alternatives that support digestion and liver detox.
- **Flaxseed and Chia Seed Substitutes**: Use oat flour, mashed bananas, or unsweetened applesauce in baking recipes where you need moisture and binding agents that seeds typically provide.

Example Recipe Modification:

- **Nut-Free Energy Balls**
  Instead of using almonds or cashews, try making energy balls with rolled oats, sunflower butter, shredded coconut, and a touch of honey. These ingredients are all liver-friendly, providing healthy fats, fiber, and a natural sweetness without the risk of allergic reactions.

4. Low-Sugar and Diabetic-Friendly Modifications

Managing blood sugar levels is a crucial part of maintaining liver health, especially for those with fatty liver disease or insulin resistance. A low-sugar or diabetic-friendly version of your favorite recipes can help prevent blood sugar spikes and ensure steady insulin production, which is key for liver detoxification and repair.

How to modify recipes:

- **Sugar Substitutes**: Use natural sweeteners such as stevia, monk fruit, or erythritol instead of refined sugar. These sweeteners have little to no impact on blood sugar and can be used in desserts, smoothies, and baked goods.
- **Fruit Alternatives**: While fruit is an excellent source of antioxidants and vitamins, certain fruits like bananas, grapes, and pineapples are higher in sugar. Opt for low-sugar fruits like berries, green apples, or kiwi for recipes where you want a touch of sweetness without the sugar spike.
- **Low-Carb Options**: For those following a low-carb or ketogenic diet, you can swap high-carb ingredients like potatoes, rice, and bread for cauliflower rice, zucchini noodles, or almond flour-based alternatives.

Example Recipe Modification:

- **Low-Sugar Berry Crumble**
Use a combination of almond flour, oats, and stevia for the crumble topping, paired with fresh mixed berries like raspberries and blackberries (which are lower in sugar) for a dessert that's both satisfying and blood-sugar friendly.

5. Anti-Inflammatory Modifications

Chronic inflammation plays a significant role in the development and progression of fatty liver disease. Incorporating anti-inflammatory foods into your liver-friendly diet can help reduce inflammation and support liver healing. Many of the ingredients used in these recipes naturally contain anti-inflammatory properties.

How to modify recipes:

- **Turmeric and Ginger**: Add turmeric and ginger to soups, smoothies, or teas. Both are natural anti-inflammatory agents that can help reduce liver inflammation and promote detoxification.
- **Leafy Greens and Cruciferous Vegetables**: Include more dark leafy greens like spinach, kale, and arugula, and cruciferous vegetables like broccoli, cauliflower, and Brussels sprouts. These vegetables are rich in antioxidants and compounds that support liver detoxification.

Example Recipe Modification:

- **Anti-Inflammatory Soup**
  Make a hearty soup using turmeric, ginger, kale, and carrots, along with bone broth or vegetable broth. This combination provides a potent anti-inflammatory boost that's gentle on the liver.

Chapter 5: Meal Prep Mastery for Fatty Liver Disease – Make Your Week Easy

Meal prepping is a powerful tool in managing fatty liver disease and maintaining a liver-healthy diet. By planning ahead and preparing your meals in advance, you set yourself up for success and ensure that you always have liver-friendly food at your fingertips. This chapter will guide you through the process of meal prepping, helping you save time, reduce stress, and stay on track with your fatty liver-friendly lifestyle. We'll also dive into specific strategies for preparing balanced meals that support liver detoxification, repair, and overall health.

Why Meal Prep is Essential for Liver Health

Living with fatty liver disease requires careful attention to your diet, which means that relying on takeout or last-minute meals can often lead to unhealthy choices. Many liver-friendly foods—rich in antioxidants, fiber, healthy fats, and lean proteins—take time to prepare and cook, but meal prep makes it easy to enjoy them every day.

Meal prep is essential for several reasons:

- **Consistency**: When you have meals ready to go, you're less likely to deviate from your liver-healthy eating plan, even when life gets busy or you're feeling tired.
- **Portion Control**: Prepping meals in advance ensures you're eating the right portion sizes, which can help with weight management and prevent overeating.
- **Stress Reduction**: Having meals already prepared eliminates the stress of trying to figure out what to eat

when you're hungry, ensuring you always have nourishing options available.
- **Nutrient-Rich Options**: With proper meal prep, you can ensure you're eating liver-friendly ingredients consistently, including healthy fats, fiber, lean proteins, and anti-inflammatory foods.

The Basics of Meal Prep for Fatty Liver Disease

Meal prepping doesn't have to be complicated or time-consuming. With a few basic strategies, you can set yourself up for a successful week of liver-healthy eating.

1. Plan Your Meals
Start by planning your meals for the week. A simple 3-day or 7-day plan works best, and don't forget to incorporate breakfast, lunch, dinner, and snacks into your prep. Here's how to structure your meals:

- **Breakfast**: Include options that are rich in fiber and healthy fats to support liver detoxification and keep you energized. Examples: smoothies, overnight oats, chia pudding, or scrambled eggs with spinach.
- **Lunch and Dinner**: Focus on balanced meals with lean proteins (chicken, turkey, fish), healthy fats (avocado, olive oil, nuts), and plenty of fiber from vegetables and whole grains. Example meals: grilled salmon with quinoa and steamed broccoli, or a turkey and avocado salad with olive oil dressing.
- **Snacks**: Pre-pack healthy snacks that you can grab on the go. Include snacks that balance blood sugar and are

rich in nutrients, such as nuts, veggies with hummus, or fruit with a handful of seeds.

2. Choose Liver-Healthy Ingredients

Be sure to incorporate ingredients that are known to support liver health, such as:

- **Leafy Greens**: Spinach, kale, arugula, and swiss chard are high in antioxidants and help detoxify the liver.
- **Cruciferous Vegetables**: Broccoli, cauliflower, and Brussels sprouts are loaded with compounds that help the liver detoxify and break down fats.
- **Healthy Fats**: Include sources of healthy fats like olive oil, avocado, and fatty fish (salmon, sardines) that provide omega-3 fatty acids for reducing inflammation in the liver.
- **Lean Proteins**: Chicken, turkey, and fish provide the protein needed for tissue repair without adding excess fat to the liver.
- **Whole Grains**: Quinoa, brown rice, and oats are high in fiber, which helps improve liver function and support digestion.

3. Organize Your Prep Day

Set aside a specific time each week—typically on a weekend day or your day off—to prep your meals. This will allow you to set yourself up for a stress-free week. During your prep day:

- **Cook in Bulk**: Prepare large batches of meals that can be easily divided into individual servings for the week. For example, cook a big batch of quinoa, rice, or roasted vegetables, and then portion them into containers.

- **Batch Cooking Proteins**: Grill, bake, or sauté your protein sources (chicken, fish, turkey) in bulk. You can then add them to salads, wraps, or grain bowls throughout the week.
- **Chop Veggies**: Pre-chop your vegetables for easy access. Keep raw veggies ready for salads, stir-fries, or snacking. You can also roast veggies in large batches and store them for quick meals.
- **Portion Your Snacks**: Portion out your snacks into small containers or bags. Pre-pack servings of nuts, seeds, hummus with veggies, or fruit so that you have them ready to go.

4. Invest in the Right Storage Containers
The key to successful meal prep is organization. Invest in high-quality glass or BPA-free plastic containers that are microwave-safe and airtight. Choose containers in various sizes for different types of meals (single servings, larger entrees, salads, etc.), and consider getting ones with compartments to separate different foods within one meal.

Meal Prep Strategies for Fatty Liver Disease

1. Batch Cooking for the Week
Cooking in bulk is one of the most efficient ways to meal prep. This allows you to have meals ready to go without needing to cook from scratch every day. Here are a few examples of batch-cooked items you can prepare:

- **Grilled Chicken Breast or Turkey**: Cook several chicken breasts or turkey fillets on a grill or in the oven.

Slice them for use in salads, wraps, or served with vegetables.
- **Quinoa, Brown Rice, or Farro**: Cook large batches of whole grains that can be used throughout the week as a base for grain bowls or as a side dish. These grains are high in fiber and have a low glycemic index, making them great for supporting liver health.
- **Roasted Vegetables**: Roast a big tray of vegetables like cauliflower, sweet potatoes, carrots, and Brussels sprouts. These can be served as sides or incorporated into salads and bowls.
- **Salmon or Sardines**: Fatty fish like salmon and sardines are great sources of omega-3 fatty acids, which are beneficial for reducing liver inflammation. Bake or grill several pieces of salmon at once for the week.

2. Pre-Making Sauces and Dressings

Liver-healthy dressings and sauces can really elevate your meals without added sugars or unhealthy fats. Making your own salad dressings and sauces in advance will save time during the week and ensure you're getting a liver-boosting flavor. Here are a few ideas:

- **Olive Oil and Lemon Vinaigrette**: Combine olive oil, lemon juice, garlic, and Dijon mustard for a tangy dressing.
- **Avocado Cilantro Dressing**: Blend avocado, cilantro, lime juice, and olive oil for a creamy dressing packed with healthy fats.
- **Turmeric Tahini Sauce**: Mix tahini, lemon juice, turmeric, and water for an anti-inflammatory, creamy dressing or dip.

3. Pre-Pack Breakfast Options

Breakfast is one of the easiest meals to prep in advance. Try these ideas:

- **Overnight Oats**: Layer rolled oats with almond milk, chia seeds, and a bit of honey in mason jars. Add berries or nuts on top for added texture.
- **Chia Pudding**: Make a batch of chia pudding using coconut milk or almond milk and let it set overnight. Top with fresh fruit or coconut flakes.
- **Smoothie Packs**: Portion out ingredients for smoothies in freezer bags. Include greens (like spinach or kale), fruits (berries, bananas), and protein powder or flaxseed. In the morning, simply blend with almond milk or water.

4. Pre-Pack Lunch and Dinner

Lunch and dinner require a bit more attention to variety, but with some planning, you can prep your meals for the week:

- **Liver-Friendly Grain Bowls**: Create grain bowls with quinoa or brown rice, roasted vegetables, and grilled chicken or salmon. Add a drizzle of olive oil and a squeeze of lemon for flavor.
- **Salads in a Jar**: Layer salad ingredients in mason jars, starting with the dressing at the bottom and ending with the greens at the top. When ready to eat, simply shake and enjoy!
- **Wraps and Burritos**: Prepare liver-friendly wraps using whole grain tortillas, lean proteins, vegetables, and healthy fats like avocado. These can be wrapped tightly and stored in the fridge for quick meals.

Meal Prep Tips for Success

1. **Keep It Simple**: Don't overcomplicate your meals. Stick with simple, whole foods that are easy to prepare, like roasted vegetables, grilled meats, and salads.
2. **Double the Recipe**: If you're already cooking a meal, double it to make extra servings that you can freeze for later.
3. **Label Your Meals**: To stay organized, label your containers with the date and meal name to ensure you eat them in order of freshness.
4. **Incorporate Leftovers**: Repurpose leftovers to avoid food waste. For example, leftover chicken can be added to a salad, while extra roasted vegetables can be incorporated into a stir-fry.
5. **Stay Flexible**: Life happens, and sometimes meal prep plans need to be adjusted. Be flexible and use what you have on hand to make meals that are still liver-healthy.

How to Meal Prep for Success: A Step-by-Step Guide to a Liver-Healthy Week

Meal prepping for the entire week may seem daunting at first, but with a little planning and organization, it can be a simple and stress-free process that helps support liver health. Meal prep ensures that you have nourishing, liver-friendly meals available at all times, reducing the temptation to resort to unhealthy, processed foods. In this guide, we will break down a step-by-step plan for meal prepping for the week, along with essential tips for creating a fatty liver-friendly grocery list to support your liver's detoxification and healing.

Step 1: Plan Your Meals for the Week

Before heading to the kitchen, the first step is to plan your meals. A well-thought-out meal plan sets the foundation for your week. Here's how to do it:

1.1 Choose Your Meals

Focus on meals that are rich in healthy fats, high in fiber, and packed with lean proteins. You'll want to choose meals that promote liver detoxification and repair, such as:

- **Breakfast**: Smoothies with spinach, berries, chia seeds, and flaxseed, or overnight oats with almond butter and nuts.
- **Lunch and Dinner**: Dishes that feature lean proteins (like chicken, turkey, or salmon), whole grains (quinoa, brown rice, or farro), and plenty of colorful vegetables (broccoli, kale, and spinach).
- **Snacks**: Nutrient-dense snacks like mixed nuts, veggie sticks with hummus, or chia pudding.

1.2 Plan for Variety

Variety is key for ensuring that you get a wide array of nutrients that benefit liver health. Choose a mix of different protein sources (fish, chicken, legumes) and rotate your vegetables and grains to keep things exciting.

1.3 Consider Meal Timing

Think about how you want to structure your meals throughout the day:

- **Breakfast**: Something quick and easy that you can grab in the morning, like smoothies or overnight oats.
- **Lunch**: A more substantial meal, like a grain bowl or a large salad with lean protein and healthy fats.
- **Dinner**: Lighter yet filling meals, such as grilled fish with roasted vegetables or a vegetable stir-fry with quinoa.
- **Snacks**: Healthy, balanced snacks to keep your energy levels steady throughout the day.

1.4 Set Realistic Portions

Portion control is important for liver health. Overeating can lead to weight gain, which strains liver function. Measure out portions and avoid using large plates that encourage overeating. Consider using smaller containers for your meals and snacks.

Step 2: Create a Fatty Liver-Friendly Grocery List

A liver-healthy grocery list is essential for meal prep success. The right ingredients will support liver function, help with weight loss, and prevent further liver damage. Here's a breakdown of what to include:

2.1 Protein Sources

Protein is crucial for the liver's repair and detox processes. Opt for lean proteins that are low in saturated fats and rich in nutrients. Some options include:

- **Fish**: Salmon, sardines, mackerel, and other fatty fish are rich in omega-3 fatty acids that reduce liver inflammation.
- **Poultry**: Skinless chicken and turkey are excellent sources of lean protein.
- **Legumes**: Beans, lentils, and chickpeas are plant-based proteins that are high in fiber and beneficial for liver function.
- **Tofu and Tempeh**: Plant-based alternatives to meat that are rich in protein and low in fat.

2.2 Healthy Fats

Healthy fats are vital for liver health, as they help reduce inflammation and support cell function. Stock up on:

- **Avocados**: High in healthy monounsaturated fats and antioxidants.
- **Olive Oil**: Rich in anti-inflammatory properties, perfect for cooking or dressings.
- **Nuts and Seeds**: Almonds, walnuts, chia seeds, and flaxseeds are full of omega-3 fatty acids and fiber.
- **Fatty Fish**: As mentioned earlier, omega-3-rich fish like salmon and sardines provide essential fats for liver health.

2.3 Vegetables

Vegetables provide antioxidants, vitamins, and fiber that support liver detoxification. Aim for a variety of colorful vegetables to maximize nutrients. Good choices include:

- **Leafy Greens**: Spinach, kale, and arugula are rich in antioxidants and help flush out toxins from the liver.
- **Cruciferous Vegetables**: Broccoli, cauliflower, Brussels sprouts, and cabbage are high in compounds that aid liver detoxification.
- **Allium Vegetables**: Garlic, onions, and leeks contain sulfur compounds that support liver enzyme function.
- **Root Vegetables**: Sweet potatoes and carrots provide fiber and vitamin A, which supports liver function.

2.4 Whole Grains

Whole grains are high in fiber, which helps regulate blood sugar and prevent fat accumulation in the liver. Include:

- **Brown Rice**: A great source of fiber and magnesium.
- **Quinoa**: A complete protein and high in antioxidants.
- **Oats**: Excellent for breakfast options like overnight oats or chia pudding.
- **Farro**: A nutrient-dense ancient grain that pairs well with vegetables and protein.

2.5 Fruits

Fruits are packed with antioxidants, vitamins, and fiber, all of which support liver health. Aim for a variety of fruits, such as:

- **Berries**: Blueberries, strawberries, and raspberries are rich in antioxidants that help fight oxidative stress.
- **Citrus Fruits**: Lemons, limes, and grapefruits are excellent for detoxifying the liver.
- **Apples**: High in pectin, which helps with toxin elimination.

2.6 Herbs and Spices

Herbs and spices are powerful anti-inflammatory ingredients that add flavor and support liver health. Include:

- **Turmeric**: Contains curcumin, which reduces inflammation and helps with liver detox.
- **Ginger**: Reduces liver inflammation and promotes digestion.
- **Cilantro**: Known for its detoxifying properties, especially for heavy metals.
- **Parsley**: Supports liver detoxification and helps reduce bloating.

2.7 Dairy Alternatives

If you're lactose intolerant or following a dairy-free diet, choose dairy alternatives like:

- **Almond Milk**: A low-calorie, calcium-rich milk alternative.
- **Coconut Yogurt**: A dairy-free option rich in probiotics that supports gut health.

Step 3: Organize and Prep Your Ingredients

With your grocery list in hand, it's time to get organized. Follow these tips for a smooth and efficient meal prep process:

3.1 Clean and Chop Ingredients

Start by washing and prepping your fruits and vegetables. Chop them into bite-sized pieces, so they're ready to go when it's time to cook. Prepping ahead saves time during the week, making it easier to assemble meals quickly.

3.2 Cook in Batches

Cooking in large batches is an efficient way to meal prep. Try these strategies:

- **Proteins**: Grill, bake, or sauté several servings of chicken, fish, or legumes. Store them in airtight containers to use throughout the week.
- **Grains**: Cook a large batch of quinoa or brown rice and store it in the fridge for easy access.
- **Vegetables**: Roast or steam vegetables in bulk, then divide them into containers.
- **Snacks**: Portion out snacks like nuts or veggie sticks with hummus into small containers for easy grab-and-go options.

3.3 Assemble Meals

Once your ingredients are prepped, start assembling your meals. You can create lunch and dinner bowls with grains, proteins, and vegetables, or prepare salads that can be dressed and eaten throughout the week. If you're prepping for breakfast, store your overnight oats or chia pudding in mason jars for easy access.

3.4 Use Containers

Invest in quality, stackable containers that make it easy to store meals. Use smaller containers for snacks, and larger ones for full meals. Label each container with the date and meal name for easy identification.

Step 4: Store and Reheat Properly

Proper storage and reheating are key to keeping your meals fresh and nutrient-dense.

4.1 Refrigeration and Freezing

- **Refrigerate** meals that you'll eat within 3-4 days.
- **Freeze** meals that are meant to be eaten later in the week. Many cooked proteins, grains, and vegetables freeze well, so make the most of your prep efforts.

4.2 Reheat with Care

Reheat your meals gently, either on the stovetop or in the microwave. Avoid overcooking, as this can degrade the nutritional value of the food. Reheat only what you need to avoid reheating and cooling food multiple times.

How to Store and Reheat Your Liver-Healthy Meals: Best Practices for Maximum Nutrient Retention

When it comes to meal prepping for a liver-healthy lifestyle, the way you store and reheat your meals is just as important as the ingredients themselves. Proper storage techniques preserve the quality and nutrients of your food, ensuring that your liver-friendly meals remain fresh, delicious, and nutritious throughout the week. In this section, we'll explore the best practices for storing and reheating your meals while maintaining the maximum nutritional value, so your liver benefits from every bite.

1. Best Practices for Storing Liver-Healthy Meals

Proper storage helps retain the nutrients in your liver-friendly meals, especially antioxidants, healthy fats, and vitamins, which can be compromised by improper handling. Let's dive into some of the top tips for storing meals and ingredients effectively.

1.1 Use Airtight Containers

Invest in high-quality, **airtight containers** to store your meals. These containers prevent air from entering, which helps to preserve freshness, texture, and nutritional content. Glass containers are especially recommended because they don't leach chemicals and tend to retain food's flavor and nutrients better than plastic.

Key Benefits:

- Airtight seals prevent moisture and air from degrading food.
- They minimize bacterial growth and help preserve vitamins and minerals.
- Glass is non-toxic and can be heated directly, reducing the risk of chemicals leaching into your food.

1.2 Store in Single-Serving Portions

Storing food in **individual portions** is a great way to avoid unnecessary reheating and help maintain optimal freshness. When you only reheat what you need, you avoid the repeated heating and cooling of your food, which can lead to nutrient loss and changes in texture.

How to do it:

- Prepare meals in single-serving containers, especially for lunch or dinner.
- Divide grains, vegetables, proteins, and snacks into separate containers, so you can easily grab and go without reheating the entire batch.

1.3 Refrigeration vs. Freezing: Know the Difference

Deciding whether to refrigerate or freeze your liver-healthy meals is essential for retaining nutrients. Here's how to store your meals based on how soon you plan to consume them:

- **Refrigeration**: Most cooked meals can be stored in the fridge for **3-4 days**. This includes proteins (chicken, fish, lean meats), cooked grains, vegetables, and salads without dressings. Refrigerating your meals helps keep

their flavors intact and slows down the growth of harmful bacteria.
- **Freezing**: If you're meal prepping for longer periods, freezing is your best option. Most cooked foods can be frozen for **up to 3 months** without significant loss in nutrient quality. You can freeze portions of soups, stews, casseroles, cooked grains, and even cooked proteins like chicken and fish.

Best Freezing Practices:

- Use **freezer-safe containers** or **zip-top bags** to store your meals. Make sure to squeeze out as much air as possible to prevent freezer burn.
- If you're freezing a large batch, portion it out into smaller, individual servings to make defrosting easier.

1.4 Store Ingredients Separately

When storing meals that will have different textures or require different reheating times (like salads with dressing, grains with sauces, or cooked protein with fresh veggies), **store the components separately**. This will help maintain the freshness and texture of each component.

For example:

- **Salads**: Store greens and dressings in separate containers. Add the dressing just before serving to prevent wilting.
- **Grains and Proteins**: Store your cooked grains and proteins in separate containers so they can be reheated according to individual needs.

1.5 Label and Date Your Meals

Always **label your containers** with the contents and the date they were made. This helps you keep track of how long meals have been stored and ensures you consume them within a safe timeframe.

How to label:

- Use a **masking tape** or **sticky notes** to label each container.
- Write the **meal name**, the **date**, and any special instructions (e.g., "reheat in microwave for 2 minutes").

2. How to Reheat Liver-Healthy Meals While Retaining Nutrients

Reheating meals correctly is crucial for maintaining the integrity of the nutrients in your liver-friendly food. Improper reheating can lead to the loss of heat-sensitive vitamins (like vitamin C) and healthy fats (like omega-3s), as well as alter the texture and flavor of your food. Here are the best methods for reheating liver-healthy meals:

2.1 Reheat with Low and Slow Heat

Avoid reheating your meals at high temperatures. Instead, opt for **low and slow heat** to preserve the integrity of nutrients and maintain a soft, appealing texture. Overheating food can cause the breakdown of essential nutrients and create an unappetizing texture.

How to reheat:

- Use **medium heat** on the stove to reheat your meals, stirring occasionally to ensure even warmth.
- When reheating in the **microwave**, use the **defrost or low heat setting** and stir the food halfway through to ensure even heating. You can also cover your food with a damp paper towel to retain moisture and prevent it from drying out.
- If using the **oven**, set it to a low temperature (about 275-300°F) to slowly reheat your meals, which helps retain the nutritional value.

2.2 Reheat Proteins Properly

Lean proteins like chicken, fish, and turkey can dry out quickly if reheated improperly, which reduces their appeal and quality. Here's how to keep your proteins moist and flavorful:

- **Chicken**: Reheat with a little **broth** or **water** in the pan or microwave. This will help keep the meat tender and juicy.
- **Fish**: Fish tends to lose moisture when reheated, so it's best to reheat in the **oven** wrapped in foil or on the stove in a covered pan. If using the microwave, reheat on low and check frequently to avoid overcooking.
- **Turkey**: Like chicken, turkey can dry out quickly. Add a splash of **broth** or cover it with a damp paper towel when microwaving.

2.3 Preserve Healthy Fats

Healthy fats, like those from **avocados**, **olive oil**, or **omega-3-rich fish**, are sensitive to heat. Overheating can cause these fats to oxidize, which diminishes their health benefits. To preserve these fats:

- **Olive oil**: Reheat food with olive oil on **low heat** to prevent the oil from breaking down.
- **Avocados**: Add fresh **avocado slices** to your meals after reheating them to preserve their nutrients.
- **Fatty fish**: When reheating fatty fish (like salmon), use a **gentle reheating method** to prevent the delicate oils from breaking down.

2.4 Reheat with Moisture

To prevent your meals from drying out during reheating, always add a bit of **moisture** to your food. This is especially important for grains, vegetables, and proteins.

Reheat tips:

- For **grains** (like quinoa, brown rice, or farro), add a spoonful of **broth** or water and cover the container when reheating to steam the food.
- **Vegetables** can be reheated with a splash of **water** or broth to prevent them from becoming rubbery or overly dry.
- When reheating **soups or stews**, keep a small amount of liquid on hand to adjust the consistency after reheating.

2.5 Avoid Reheating Multiple Times

To preserve the nutritional value of your food, **avoid reheating meals more than once**. Every time food is reheated and cooled, its nutrient content diminishes, especially vitamins like vitamin C and folate. If you have leftovers, consider using them in a different meal, or store them in the fridge or freezer to use in the coming days.

3. Quick Tips for Meal Storage and Reheating Success

- **Keep it airtight**: Always use airtight containers to preserve freshness and reduce the risk of spoilage.
- **Don't overcook**: Avoid overcooking or reheating your meals at high temperatures, as this can lead to nutrient loss.
- **Portion out meals**: Store meals in individual portions to avoid multiple reheating sessions, which can degrade food quality.
- **Label meals**: Label each container with the date of preparation to ensure you eat your meals within the safe storage window.
- **Reheat slowly**: Reheat your food slowly and with moisture to retain nutrients and texture.

Batch Cooking Techniques: Save Time and Stick to Your Diet with Efficient Cooking Strategies

Batch cooking is a game-changer when it comes to maintaining a liver-healthy lifestyle. It allows you to prepare large quantities of food at once, saving you time during the week and making it easier to stay on track with your diet. With the right strategies, batch cooking can streamline your meal preparation, ensure you have liver-friendly options ready when you need them, and help you avoid unhealthy temptations.

In this section, we'll explore the art of batch cooking—how to do it efficiently, what foods are ideal for batch cooking, and how to store and reheat your meals without losing nutrients. Whether you're meal prepping for the entire week or just making enough food for a few days, batch cooking can make sticking to your fatty liver-friendly diet both convenient and sustainable.

1. Benefits of Batch Cooking for Liver Health

Before we dive into the how-to, let's take a look at why batch cooking is such a powerful tool in the fight against fatty liver disease.

1.1 Saves Time and Effort

Batch cooking allows you to prepare meals in bulk, reducing the need to cook every day. Once you've cooked large quantities of food, you can store it in the fridge or freezer and reheat it when needed. This eliminates the need for daily cooking, which can be time-consuming, especially when following a strict, liver-healthy diet.

1.2 Reduces Stress Around Meal Time

Having pre-prepared meals available makes it easier to avoid the stress of deciding what to eat every day. Batch cooking takes the guesswork out of meal planning, helping you stay focused on your health goals without the temptation to reach for unhealthy options.

1.3 Ensures Consistency

Batch cooking ensures that you always have liver-healthy meals on hand, preventing you from resorting to quick, unhealthy options or dining out. It gives you greater control over the quality and nutritional content of your food.

1.4 Supports Long-Term Health Goals

By sticking to a meal prep routine, you are consistently feeding your body with the right nutrients that support liver detox, improve insulin sensitivity, and fight inflammation—all essential components of reversing and preventing fatty liver disease.

2. How to Batch Cook Effectively

The key to successful batch cooking is planning and organization. By following these steps, you'll be able to prepare liver-friendly meals that will stay fresh, nutritious, and easy to access throughout the week.

2.1 Plan Your Meals in Advance

Start by selecting recipes that are **liver-friendly** and can be made in large batches. Plan your meals around whole foods, high-fiber vegetables, lean proteins, healthy fats, and low-glycemic carbohydrates. This ensures that all the nutrients your liver needs are included, and you can easily integrate these meals into your diet.

Meal Planning Tips:

- Plan meals for **5-7 days** in advance.
- Include **variety** to prevent boredom. For example, make different types of grain bowls, salads, or vegetable stews throughout the week.
- **Balance your meals**: Aim for meals that combine healthy fats (e.g., avocado, olive oil, omega-3-rich fish), lean proteins (e.g., chicken, tofu, lentils), and complex carbs (e.g., quinoa, sweet potatoes).

2.2 Make a Shopping List

Once you've planned your meals, create a shopping list based on the ingredients you'll need. Having a list ensures you won't forget key items and helps streamline the shopping process. It also minimizes impulse buys, making it easier to stick to your healthy eating plan.

Shopping List Tips:

- **Organize by food category**: Group items by sections like produce, proteins, grains, and pantry essentials to save time while shopping.
- **Buy in bulk**: Purchase whole grains, beans, and vegetables in bulk, as these are often cheaper and store well for extended periods.
- **Choose fresh and frozen**: Fresh vegetables are great, but don't forget frozen vegetables, which are often just as nutritious and can be stored longer.

2.3 Cook in Bulk

Batch cooking is about making large quantities of food at once. Focus on cooking in bulk for key ingredients like grains, proteins, and vegetables, which can be combined in various ways throughout the week.

Steps to cook in bulk:

- **Cook grains in large quantities**: Whole grains like quinoa, brown rice, and farro can be cooked in big batches and stored in the fridge for up to 5 days or frozen for later use. Make enough to last for multiple meals.
- **Prepare proteins**: Cook proteins like chicken breast, turkey, or plant-based options (tofu, tempeh) in large batches. Roast, grill, or bake them in the oven to cook efficiently and in large quantities.
- **Vegetable prep**: Roasting or steaming vegetables like broccoli, cauliflower, carrots, and sweet potatoes in large quantities is an efficient way to prep your veggies for the week. You can also chop raw veggies and store them in the fridge for salads or stir-fries.

Cooking Tips:

- Cook grains in a **rice cooker** or **instant pot** to save time and effort.
- Use a **sheet pan** for roasting multiple vegetables at once.
- **Slow cook** proteins like chicken or beef in a crockpot or instant pot to break them down into tender pieces, making them easier to add to a variety of meals.

2.4 Use One-Pot or One-Pan Meals

One-pot or one-pan meals are great for batch cooking because they allow you to cook multiple ingredients together, saving time on preparation and cleanup. Consider dishes like soups, stews, and casseroles that can be made in a large pot or a slow cooker. These dishes also tend to improve in flavor over time, making them perfect for storing and reheating.

Examples of one-pot meals:

- **Lentil and vegetable stew**: Cook a large batch of lentils, vegetables, and broth for a nutrient-rich, liver-friendly meal.
- **Quinoa and chicken stir-fry**: Combine quinoa with chicken, vegetables, and olive oil for a simple and satisfying meal that you can portion out for the week.=

3. How to Store Your Batch-Cooked Meals

Once you've cooked everything in bulk, it's time to store your meals. The key is to keep your food fresh and easy to access while maintaining its nutritional quality.

3.1 Store in Airtight Containers

As with any meal prep, use **airtight containers** to store your cooked foods. This will prevent air from entering and moisture from escaping, keeping your meals fresh longer. Glass containers are preferred because they are non-toxic and better at preserving the flavor and texture of your food.

Storage Tips:

- Use **separate containers** for proteins, grains, and vegetables, so you can mix and match meals as needed.
- Store **individual portions** to make it easier to grab a meal or reheat only what you need.
- Label each container with the **date** it was cooked, so you know when to consume it.

3.2 Freeze for Longer Storage

If you want to prepare meals for several weeks, freezing your batch-cooked meals is the way to go. Most dishes, including grains, proteins, and even soups and stews, can be frozen for **up to 3 months** without significant nutrient loss.

Freezing Tips:

- Let food **cool** to room temperature before freezing to prevent condensation and ice crystals from forming.
- Use **freezer-safe bags or containers** and squeeze out any air to avoid freezer burn.
- **Portion out meals** into single-serving sizes before freezing for easy reheating.

3.3 Refrigeration for Quick Access

If you plan to eat your batch-cooked meals within the week, refrigerating them is your best option. Most cooked meals will last in the fridge for **3-5 days**, and the convenience of having meals ready to go can help you stay on track with your liver-healthy diet.

4. How to Reheat Batch-Cooked Meals Without Losing Nutrients

Reheating your pre-cooked meals is an essential part of the process, but you must do it properly to ensure the food retains its nutritional value.

Reheating Tips:

- Reheat meals at **low heat** to prevent overcooking and preserve the nutrients.
- Use **moisture** (like broth or water) when reheating grains or proteins to prevent them from drying out.
- When using the **microwave**, cover the food with a damp paper towel to keep it moist and heat evenly.

Chapter 6: Understanding Liver Detox – What Your Liver Really Needs

The liver is one of the hardest-working organs in your body, performing over 500 essential functions, including detoxification, metabolism, protein synthesis, and the production of bile. Its primary role is to filter toxins from the blood and process nutrients, helping to maintain the body's balance. However, over time, the liver can become overwhelmed by the toxins and excess fat that accumulate due to poor lifestyle habits, improper diet, or environmental factors. This chapter delves into the science of liver detoxification, explaining what your liver needs to function optimally and how you can support it naturally.

1. The Liver's Detoxification Process: How It Works

The liver's detoxification process is a complex, multi-stage operation designed to neutralize and eliminate harmful substances from the body. The liver uses a two-phase system to metabolize and excrete toxins—whether they come from food, alcohol, environmental pollutants, or internal byproducts of metabolism.

1.1 Phase 1: Breaking Down Toxins

Phase 1 of liver detoxification involves breaking down toxins into smaller, more water-soluble molecules. This process is carried out by enzymes, primarily the **cytochrome P450 enzyme system**, which works to modify toxic substances by oxidizing or reducing them. These substances are then made more reactive or less toxic, but some may become temporarily more harmful.

Important enzymes involved:

- **CYP450 enzymes**: Break down and metabolize toxins, including chemicals from medications, alcohol, and pesticides.
- **NADPH**: Provides the necessary energy for Phase 1 enzyme reactions.

While Phase 1 detoxifies substances, it can sometimes make certain chemicals more harmful, creating intermediate compounds. This is why Phase 2 is crucial for processing these toxins further.

1.2 Phase 2: Conjugation and Elimination

In Phase 2, the liver cells conjugate (bind) these intermediate toxins to other molecules to neutralize them and make them easier to eliminate through the urine or bile. This phase involves various detoxification pathways, including **glutathione conjugation, sulfation, glucuronidation,** and **acetylation.**

- **Glutathione**: This antioxidant is one of the most important molecules in Phase 2 detoxification. It binds with toxins to neutralize them and prevent them from causing oxidative damage.
- **Sulfation and Glucuronidation**: These pathways attach sulfate or glucuronic acid to toxins, making them more water-soluble and easier to excrete.

Once the toxins are neutralized and bound, they can then be safely eliminated from the body through bile, which is excreted into the intestines, or through the kidneys in the urine.

2. The Importance of Supporting the Liver's Detoxification

The liver detoxification process is essential for maintaining overall health, as it filters out harmful substances that could otherwise accumulate and cause disease. However, the liver can become overburdened when it faces an overwhelming number of toxins. This is where liver support becomes crucial.

2.1 The Role of Antioxidants in Liver Detox

Antioxidants, such as **vitamin C**, **vitamin E**, and **selenium**, play an important role in neutralizing free radicals and oxidative stress that can arise during the liver's detoxification processes. They help protect liver cells from damage caused by the breakdown of toxins and promote cellular repair.

In addition, antioxidants **regenerate** glutathione, one of the liver's most vital detoxifying agents, ensuring its continued function in both Phase 1 and Phase 2 detoxification.

2.2 Supporting Enzyme Activity

The liver's detoxification enzymes need proper nutrients and cofactors to function optimally. Key nutrients that support liver detox include:

- **B Vitamins** (especially B6, B12, and folate): These are crucial for enzyme activity, especially in Phase 1 detox.
- **Magnesium**: Supports enzymatic processes and helps regulate liver function.
- **Zinc**: A key mineral in the synthesis of liver enzymes, including those involved in Phase 1 detox.

2.3 The Role of Fiber in Detoxification

Fiber plays a key role in the detoxification process by binding to waste products and toxins in the intestines, promoting their elimination. A diet high in **soluble and insoluble fiber** helps support liver function by reducing the burden of detoxification on the liver.

- **Soluble fiber**, found in foods like oats, apples, and beans, binds with cholesterol and toxins to carry them out of the body through the digestive tract.
- **Insoluble fiber**, found in foods like vegetables, whole grains, and seeds, helps move waste efficiently through the intestines and supports the detoxification of liver waste.

Fiber-rich foods also regulate blood sugar levels, preventing insulin spikes that could lead to fat accumulation in the liver, a key factor in fatty liver disease.

3. Foods That Promote Liver Detoxification

Eating the right foods can help nourish your liver, promote detoxification, and reduce the risk of fatty liver disease. Many foods contain specific compounds and nutrients that support liver function, combat oxidative stress, and aid in toxin elimination.

3.1 Cruciferous Vegetables

Cruciferous vegetables like **broccoli**, **cauliflower**, **Brussels sprouts**, and **kale** are rich in **sulfur-containing compounds** (such as glucosinolates) that enhance Phase 2 detoxification. These compounds support the liver's ability to neutralize toxins, making them essential for liver health.

3.2 Leafy Greens and Bitter Vegetables

Leafy greens, such as **spinach**, **arugula**, and **dandelion greens**, as well as bitter vegetables like **artichokes**, promote bile production and support the liver's detox pathways. They help flush out toxins through the bile and stimulate healthy digestion.

3.3 Garlic and Onions

Garlic and onions contain sulfur compounds (like allicin and diallyl disulfide) that support liver enzymes involved in detoxification. These compounds also promote the production of glutathione, one of the liver's key detoxifiers.

3.4 Beets and Carrots

Beets and carrots are rich in **beta-carotene** and **antioxidants**, which help protect liver cells from oxidative damage. Beets, in particular, help stimulate the liver's detox pathways and improve bile production, aiding in toxin elimination.

3.5 Fatty Fish (Omega-3 Fatty Acids)

Fatty fish, such as **salmon, mackerel**, and **sardines**, are high in **omega-3 fatty acids**, which help reduce liver fat and inflammation. Omega-3s also support the liver's ability to metabolize fats and reduce oxidative stress.

3.6 Turmeric

Turmeric contains **curcumin**, a powerful anti-inflammatory compound that promotes bile production and enhances liver detoxification. Curcumin has been shown to protect the liver from damage caused by toxins and inflammation, supporting its ability to clear out waste.

3.7 Green Tea

Green tea is rich in **catechins**, antioxidants that have been shown to support liver function and reduce the risk of fatty liver disease. Regular consumption of green tea has been associated with improved liver enzyme levels and overall liver health.

4. Lifestyle Changes to Support Liver Detox

In addition to consuming liver-friendly foods, certain lifestyle changes can enhance liver detoxification and improve overall liver health.

4.1 Staying Hydrated

Drinking plenty of water is essential for liver detoxification. Water helps the liver flush out toxins through the kidneys and maintains optimal liver function. Aim for at least 8 cups of water daily, and more if you're physically active or live in a hot climate.

4.2 Regular Exercise

Exercise plays a vital role in maintaining a healthy liver. Physical activity improves circulation, reduces insulin resistance, and helps with weight management, all of which are important for preventing and reversing fatty liver disease. Aim for **30 minutes of moderate exercise** (like walking, cycling, or swimming) at least 5 days a week.

4.3 Getting Enough Sleep

Quality sleep is crucial for liver function. The liver performs many of its detoxification processes during sleep, including the synthesis of key enzymes and the processing of waste. Aim for **7-9 hours of quality sleep** each night to support liver health.

5. The Bottom Line: Supporting Liver Detoxification for Better Health

The liver is an incredible organ capable of detoxifying and healing itself. However, when faced with excessive toxins, poor diet, and environmental stressors, it can become overloaded, which may contribute to liver diseases like fatty liver. Supporting liver detoxification through a nutrient-dense diet, hydration, regular exercise, and lifestyle changes can help prevent liver damage, reduce inflammation, and enhance detoxification.

By understanding the science behind liver detox and nourishing your body with the right foods and habits, you can significantly improve your liver health and give it the support it needs to function at its best.

The Truth About Detoxing: How the Liver Detoxifies Naturally and How You Can Support This Process

When it comes to detoxification, the liver is the body's unsung hero. While detox programs and cleanses are often marketed as essential for purging toxins, the truth is that your liver is already hard at work detoxifying your body every day—naturally, without the need for expensive supplements or fad diets. The liver is a powerful, self-regulating organ with a remarkable ability to process and eliminate harmful substances. However, certain lifestyle factors can strain its detoxification capacity, leading to the accumulation of toxins and the development of conditions like fatty liver disease. In this chapter, we'll uncover how the liver detoxifies naturally, explore the myths surrounding detox programs, and discuss how you can support this vital process with simple, evidence-based strategies.

1. How the Liver Detoxifies Naturally: The Science Behind It

The liver is the body's primary detoxification organ. It processes all blood that comes from the digestive tract, making it a key player in removing harmful substances, balancing nutrients, and maintaining the body's overall health. The detoxification process in the liver involves multiple phases, primarily aimed at neutralizing or eliminating toxins so they no longer pose a risk to the body.

1.1 Phase 1: Breaking Down Toxins

The first stage of detoxification occurs when the liver breaks down fat-soluble toxins into water-soluble compounds. This is done through a system of enzymes, most notably the **cytochrome P450 enzyme system**, which helps to metabolize drugs, alcohol, environmental toxins, and other chemicals that enter the bloodstream.

- **Cytochrome P450 Enzymes**: These enzymes transform fat-soluble toxins (like alcohol, caffeine, pesticides, and chemicals from processed foods) into more easily excreted substances. In the process, these toxins are converted into intermediate compounds that are more reactive but also easier to neutralize.

However, these intermediate compounds can be more harmful if left unchecked. That's where Phase 2 comes into play.

1.2 Phase 2: Conjugation and Neutralization

Once the toxins are broken down into intermediate compounds in Phase 1, the liver's Phase 2 enzymes conjugate these compounds with various molecules, such as **glutathione**, **sulfate**, or **glucuronic acid**, to make them water-soluble. This makes the toxins much less harmful and ensures they can be efficiently eliminated from the body through bile or urine.

- **Glutathione**: Known as the liver's "master antioxidant," glutathione binds with toxins, neutralizing their effects and supporting cellular repair in the liver. It plays a crucial role in Phase 2 detoxification, and maintaining adequate levels of glutathione is vital for liver health.
- **Conjugation**: In this process, the liver combines toxins with molecules that render them harmless and enable their easy excretion through bile (into the intestines) or urine (via the kidneys).

1.3 Elimination: The Final Step

After the liver neutralizes and conjugates toxins, they are eliminated from the body through the digestive system (in bile) or the urinary system (in urine). Bile is stored in the gallbladder and then released into the small intestine to help digest fats. Any toxins that were neutralized by the liver are excreted with the bile. Alternatively, water-soluble toxins are filtered by the kidneys and excreted in urine.

This entire process occurs continuously and efficiently when the liver is supported and not overwhelmed by excessive toxins or poor lifestyle habits.

2. Common Myths About Detoxing

Detoxing has become a buzzword in the wellness industry, with many detox products, cleanses, and fasting protocols promising to "cleanse" the body of toxins. However, these claims are often misleading or exaggerated. Let's explore some common detox myths and set the record straight.

2.1 Myth #1: You Need Expensive Detox Products to Cleanse Your Liver

One of the biggest myths is that the liver needs special products or detox programs to do its job. In reality, the liver is fully equipped to detoxify the body without the need for expensive supplements, juices, or cleanses. While some products may contain beneficial nutrients like **milk thistle**, **dandelion root**, or **turmeric**, the liver itself has evolved to handle detoxification naturally.

The truth: You don't need expensive detox programs. A balanced diet, regular hydration, and a healthy lifestyle are often enough to support the liver's detoxification abilities.

2.2 Myth #2: Fasting is the Best Way to Detoxify Your Body

Fasting is often promoted as a way to give the liver a break and jump-start detoxification. While intermittent fasting or caloric restriction may offer health benefits for some, it is not a magic solution for detoxing. In fact, overdoing fasting can strain the liver and the body's natural detox processes, especially when hydration and nutrient intake are compromised.

The truth: Instead of prolonged or extreme fasting, the body benefits from consistent, balanced eating, including foods that promote liver health and detoxification. Short, intermittent fasting can offer benefits when done mindfully, but it's not a one-size-fits-all solution.

2.3 Myth #3: Liver Detoxing Can Be Done Quickly

Many detox programs promise quick results, claiming to "cleanse" the liver in a matter of days. Detoxification is a slow and steady process that works best over time. For the liver to fully process and eliminate toxins, it requires consistent support, proper nutrition, hydration, and regular rest.

The truth: Detoxing takes time. It's a continuous, ongoing process that works best with consistent, healthy habits rather than relying on quick fixes.

3. How to Support Your Liver's Natural Detox Process

The good news is that you can help your liver work more effectively and efficiently through small, sustainable lifestyle and dietary changes. Let's look at some key ways to support your liver's natural detoxification process.

3.1 Eat a Liver-Friendly Diet

A nutrient-dense diet full of whole foods can nourish and support the liver. Focus on:

- **Antioxidant-rich foods** like **berries, green leafy vegetables**, and **cruciferous vegetables** (broccoli, cauliflower, kale) to reduce oxidative stress and help the liver neutralize toxins.
- **Healthy fats** from **avocados, nuts, seeds**, and **fatty fish** (salmon, mackerel) to provide essential fatty acids that support liver cell membranes and help with fat metabolism.

- **High-fiber foods** like **whole grains**, **vegetables**, and **fruits** that promote regular bowel movements, helping to expel toxins through the digestive system.
- **Sulfur-rich foods** like **garlic**, **onions**, and **eggs**, which help with Phase 2 detoxification pathways, improving the liver's ability to neutralize toxins.

3.2 Stay Hydrated

Drinking plenty of water is vital for liver health. Water helps flush out toxins through the kidneys, supports bile production, and ensures that waste products can be properly eliminated from the body. Aim for at least 8 cups (64 oz) of water daily.

3.3 Regular Exercise

Exercise boosts blood flow, which helps the liver deliver oxygen and nutrients more efficiently to its cells, enhancing detoxification. Physical activity also reduces fat accumulation in the liver, which is essential for maintaining optimal liver function. Aim for at least 30 minutes of moderate activity most days of the week.

3.4 Avoid Alcohol and Toxins

Excessive alcohol consumption is one of the biggest contributors to liver damage and fatty liver disease. It overloads the liver, impairing its detoxification process and causing inflammation. Reducing or eliminating alcohol intake and limiting exposure to environmental toxins (like cigarette smoke, pesticides, and chemicals) helps prevent liver stress and supports its natural detoxification pathways.

3.5 Prioritize Sleep

Your liver works hard during sleep to detoxify the body and repair damaged cells. Ensuring you get enough restful sleep (7-9 hours per night) is essential for liver health and effective detoxification. Sleep also supports the body's hormone regulation, which plays a role in liver function and fat metabolism.

4. The Bottom Line: Trust Your Liver's Natural Detox Process

The liver is an incredibly resilient organ that is fully capable of detoxifying the body without the need for external interventions. By supporting its natural detoxification process through a balanced diet, hydration, exercise, and healthy habits, you can ensure that your liver is functioning optimally. Remember, the best way to promote liver health is through consistency—sustained lifestyle changes that provide the nutrients, rest, and support the liver needs to thrive.

Rather than relying on quick-fix detox programs or cleanses, focus on long-term strategies that allow your liver to perform its natural detoxification functions. With the right habits in place, your liver will thank you by keeping your body clean, balanced, and healthy for years to come.

Natural Liver Cleansers: Foods, Herbs, and Supplements that Promote Liver Detox

The liver is one of the most vital organs in the body, serving as the primary detoxification hub. It filters and breaks down toxins, processes fats, stores vitamins and minerals, and helps regulate blood sugar levels. However, over time, the liver can become overloaded with toxins from processed foods, environmental pollutants, alcohol, and medications, potentially leading to conditions like fatty liver disease, liver inflammation, and other metabolic imbalances. While the liver is highly capable of detoxifying the body on its own, supporting it with natural liver cleansers can enhance its ability to cleanse and repair itself.

In this chapter, we'll explore the various foods, herbs, and supplements that promote liver detoxification, helping to support optimal liver function and overall health.

1. Foods that Promote Liver Detoxification

A healthy diet is one of the most effective ways to support liver function and promote detoxification. Certain foods contain specific nutrients that help the liver perform its detoxifying tasks more efficiently. Below are some of the top liver-friendly foods:

1.1 Cruciferous Vegetables (Broccoli, Brussels Sprouts, Kale, Cauliflower)

Cruciferous vegetables are rich in **sulfur compounds**, such as **glucosinolates**, which help boost the liver's Phase 2 detoxification process. These compounds enhance the liver's ability to neutralize toxins and eliminate them through bile and urine. They also contain **fiber**, which helps support digestive health and reduce the burden on the liver.

- **Benefits for the liver:** Supports detoxification, aids in fat metabolism, and reduces oxidative stress.
- **How to incorporate them:** Enjoy steamed or sautéed broccoli, kale, and cauliflower as side dishes, or add them to soups and salads.

1.2 Leafy Greens (Spinach, Swiss Chard, Dandelion Greens)

Leafy greens are packed with **chlorophyll**, which helps to detoxify the liver by neutralizing environmental toxins, pesticides, and heavy metals. Chlorophyll also enhances bile production, aiding the liver in processing and eliminating waste. Additionally, greens like **dandelion root** support liver health by stimulating bile flow and supporting liver regeneration.

- **Benefits for the liver:** Detoxifies toxins, supports bile production, and helps maintain healthy liver function.
- **How to incorporate them:** Blend leafy greens into smoothies, toss them in salads, or sauté them with garlic and olive oil.

1.3 Garlic and Onions

Both garlic and onions contain powerful compounds, such as **allicin** and **organosulfur compounds**, that support liver detoxification. These compounds help activate liver enzymes that aid in breaking down and removing toxins. Additionally, garlic contains **selenium**, an antioxidant that helps protect the liver from oxidative damage.

- **Benefits for the liver:** Stimulates liver enzymes, boosts detoxification, and provides antioxidant support.

- **How to incorporate them:** Add garlic and onions to soups, stews, salads, or roasted vegetables to enhance flavor and liver support.

1.4 Beets

Beets are rich in **betaines**, compounds that support liver function by helping the liver cells flush out toxins more effectively. Beets also stimulate bile production and enhance fat metabolism, both of which are essential for detoxification. The high fiber content in beets helps support digestion and prevent constipation, which allows for more efficient toxin elimination.

- **Benefits for the liver:** Supports liver detoxification, promotes bile production, and aids fat metabolism.
- **How to incorporate them:** Roast or steam beets, or add them raw to juices and smoothies.

1.5 Turmeric

Turmeric contains **curcumin**, a powerful anti-inflammatory and antioxidant compound that has been shown to enhance liver function by promoting the detoxification processes in the liver. Curcumin helps to reduce oxidative stress and inflammation, two factors that can impair liver function. Additionally, turmeric stimulates bile production, which aids in the digestion and removal of fats.

- **Benefits for the liver:** Reduces inflammation, enhances detoxification, and supports bile production.

- **How to incorporate it:** Add turmeric to curries, soups, teas, or smoothies. Pair it with black pepper to improve curcumin absorption.

1.6 Avocados

Avocados are packed with **healthy fats** (monounsaturated fats), particularly oleic acid, which support liver health by reducing fat buildup in the liver and promoting healthy liver cell membranes. Avocados are also rich in **glutathione**, a potent antioxidant that plays a key role in liver detoxification.

- **Benefits for the liver:** Reduces liver fat accumulation, supports healthy liver function, and provides antioxidant support.
- **How to incorporate them:** Add avocado slices to salads, spread on whole-grain toast, or blend into smoothies.

1.7 Green Tea

Green tea is loaded with **catechins**, antioxidants that support liver health by reducing fat accumulation and inflammation in the liver. Some studies suggest that regular consumption of green tea may help reduce the risk of fatty liver disease and promote liver enzyme balance.

- **Benefits for the liver:** Reduces liver fat, enhances liver function, and provides antioxidant protection.
- **How to incorporate it:** Drink 1–2 cups of green tea daily to support detoxification.

2. Herbs that Support Liver Detoxification

In addition to foods, several herbs have been shown to support liver detoxification. Many of these herbs have a long history of use in traditional medicine and have been researched for their liver-protective properties.

2.1 Milk Thistle

Milk thistle (Silybum marianum) is one of the most well-known liver herbs. The active compound, **silymarin**, is a potent antioxidant that protects the liver cells from oxidative damage and helps regenerate liver tissue. Milk thistle has been shown to support the liver in detoxifying chemicals, alcohol, and other toxins. It is also effective in reducing inflammation and promoting overall liver health.

- **Benefits for the liver:** Regenerates liver cells, reduces liver inflammation, and protects against oxidative damage.
- **How to incorporate it:** Milk thistle is commonly available in supplement form. It can be taken as a capsule, tincture, or tea.

2.2 Dandelion Root

Dandelion root is another excellent herb for supporting liver health. It helps stimulate the production of bile, which is essential for fat digestion and toxin elimination. Additionally, dandelion root has natural diuretic properties, helping to flush toxins from the body through urine.

- **Benefits for the liver:** Stimulates bile production, enhances toxin removal, and supports liver detoxification.
- **How to incorporate it:** Dandelion root can be consumed as a tea, tincture, or in capsule form.

2.3 Artichoke

Artichoke extract contains **cynarin**, a compound that supports the liver's detoxification processes by stimulating bile production. Cynarin helps the liver break down and eliminate fats, promoting digestion and supporting the liver's natural detox pathways.

- **Benefits for the liver:** Supports bile production, enhances fat digestion, and detoxifies the liver.
- **How to incorporate it:** Artichoke can be consumed as a vegetable in salads or steamed dishes. Artichoke extract is also available as a supplement.

2.4 Burdock Root

Burdock root has been used for centuries in traditional medicine for its detoxifying properties. It helps cleanse the blood and liver by promoting urination and sweating, both of which help remove toxins from the body. Burdock root also has anti-inflammatory and antioxidant properties, making it a great ally for liver health.

- **Benefits for the liver:** Promotes detoxification, reduces inflammation, and protects liver cells from oxidative stress.

- **How to incorporate it:** Burdock root can be consumed as a tea, tincture, or added to soups and stews.

3. Supplements That Support Liver Detoxification

While a healthy diet and herbal remedies are often enough to support liver detox, certain supplements can further boost liver health, especially for those with liver conditions or those who want to ensure their liver is functioning at its best.

3.1 N-Acetyl Cysteine (NAC)

N-Acetyl Cysteine (NAC) is a powerful supplement that helps increase the body's levels of **glutathione**, the liver's master antioxidant. NAC has been shown to protect the liver from damage caused by toxins, alcohol, and drugs while supporting the liver's detoxification processes.

- **Benefits for the liver:** Boosts glutathione production, protects liver cells from oxidative damage, and supports liver detoxification.
- **How to incorporate it:** NAC is available in capsule or powder form and should be taken according to recommended dosages.

3.2 Vitamin E

Vitamin E is a potent antioxidant that helps protect the liver from oxidative stress and inflammation. It has been studied for its ability to improve liver function, particularly in people with fatty liver disease.

- **Benefits for the liver:** Reduces oxidative damage, supports liver health, and improves liver function.
- **How to incorporate it:** Vitamin E is available as a supplement, or you can include more foods rich in vitamin E, such as almonds, sunflower seeds, and spinach.

3.3 Zinc

Zinc is an essential mineral that plays a crucial role in supporting the liver's detoxification enzymes. It has antioxidant and anti-inflammatory properties, and zinc deficiency can impair liver function.

- **Benefits for the liver:** Enhances liver detoxification, supports enzyme function, and reduces inflammation.
- **How to incorporate it:** Zinc supplements are widely available, or you can consume zinc-rich foods like pumpkin seeds, shellfish, and lentils.

Daily Habits to Support Liver Health

The liver is a powerhouse organ, responsible for detoxifying the body, processing nutrients, metabolizing fats, and storing vitamins and minerals. It works tirelessly behind the scenes to keep our bodies functioning properly. However, lifestyle factors such as poor diet, lack of exercise, and insufficient rest can lead to liver stress and dysfunction over time. Fortunately, adopting simple daily habits can significantly enhance liver function, support detoxification, and promote long-term liver health.

In this section, we will explore the daily habits you can incorporate into your routine to boost liver health, from staying hydrated to managing stress and getting quality sleep.

1. Stay Hydrated

Hydration is one of the most essential habits for maintaining liver health. Water plays a vital role in supporting the liver's detoxification processes. The liver requires an adequate supply of fluids to filter toxins, metabolize nutrients, and process waste. Additionally, hydration helps prevent the liver from becoming overburdened by waste buildup and ensures that toxins are flushed out effectively.

Why Hydration Matters for Liver Health:

- **Detoxification:** The liver uses water to filter out waste products and toxins from the blood, which are then excreted via urine and bile. Without sufficient water, this detoxification process can slow down.
- **Bile Production:** Adequate hydration supports the production of bile, a substance critical for fat digestion and detoxification.
- **Prevents Liver Congestion:** Staying hydrated helps prevent the liver from becoming congested with waste, reducing the risk of fatty liver and other liver-related conditions.

How to Stay Hydrated:

- **Drink Water Regularly:** Aim for at least 8 cups (2 liters) of water daily, and adjust based on your individual needs (activity level, climate, etc.).
- **Herbal Teas:** Herbal teas such as dandelion root, milk thistle, and peppermint not only hydrate but also support liver function.
- **Water-Rich Foods:** Incorporate water-rich fruits and vegetables, such as cucumbers, watermelon, and oranges, into your daily meals.

2. Exercise Regularly

Regular physical activity is another cornerstone of liver health. Exercise has numerous benefits for the liver, ranging from weight management to improved circulation, both of which are vital for optimal liver function. Physical activity helps the liver burn fat, regulate blood sugar, and promote the efficient processing of nutrients and toxins.

Why Exercise Supports Liver Health:

- **Weight Management:** Excess body fat, especially abdominal fat, is a primary contributor to **fatty liver disease**. Exercise helps reduce visceral fat, improving liver function.
- **Improved Insulin Sensitivity:** Regular exercise increases insulin sensitivity, reducing the risk of developing insulin resistance, which is linked to liver disease.

- **Enhanced Blood Circulation:** Exercise boosts blood circulation, helping the liver efficiently process toxins and nutrients.
- **Liver Regeneration:** Studies suggest that exercise supports liver regeneration by promoting the production of new liver cells.

How to Incorporate Exercise into Your Routine:

- **Cardio Workouts:** Engage in aerobic exercises such as walking, jogging, swimming, or cycling for at least 30 minutes a day. Aim for at least 5 days a week.
- **Strength Training:** Incorporate strength training exercises (weight lifting or bodyweight exercises) at least twice a week to increase muscle mass and support fat metabolism.
- **Stretching & Yoga:** Incorporate stretching or yoga into your routine to reduce stress and improve liver detoxification by promoting lymphatic drainage and circulation.

3. Prioritize Quality Sleep

Adequate, restful sleep is critical for liver health. The liver detoxifies the body, metabolizes fats, and processes hormones at night, especially during the deep stages of sleep. Poor sleep or chronic sleep deprivation can impair liver function, leading to an increased risk of fatty liver, insulin resistance, and other metabolic issues.

Why Sleep is Crucial for Liver Health:

- **Liver Repair and Detoxification:** The liver works hard to repair itself and process toxins while you sleep. Without enough rest, this detoxification process is compromised.
- **Hormonal Balance:** Sleep helps regulate the production of hormones like cortisol and insulin, which influence liver metabolism and fat storage.
- **Restores Energy Levels:** Sleep supports overall energy metabolism, allowing the liver to process and utilize nutrients more effectively.

How to Improve Sleep Quality:

- **Establish a Sleep Routine:** Go to bed and wake up at the same time every day to regulate your body's internal clock.
- **Create a Relaxing Environment:** Make your sleep environment comfortable—keep the room dark, cool, and quiet to promote deep sleep.
- **Limit Screen Time:** Avoid screens (phone, computer, TV) at least an hour before bed, as the blue light emitted can interfere with melatonin production, a hormone that helps you fall asleep.
- **Relaxation Techniques:** Practice deep breathing, meditation, or gentle yoga before bed to reduce stress and promote relaxation.

4. Eat a Liver-Healthy Diet

A balanced, nutrient-rich diet is a crucial part of any liver-supporting routine. The liver thrives on foods rich in antioxidants, healthy fats, fiber, and essential vitamins and minerals. A diet high in processed foods, sugar, and trans fats can overload the liver with toxins and cause fat buildup, leading to liver disease.

Why Diet Matters for Liver Health:

- **Supports Detoxification:** Nutrient-dense foods like fruits, vegetables, and whole grains provide the necessary vitamins, minerals, and antioxidants that support liver detoxification.
- **Reduces Inflammation:** A healthy diet rich in anti-inflammatory foods, such as omega-3 fatty acids from fish or flaxseeds, can help reduce liver inflammation and oxidative stress.
- **Promotes Fat Metabolism:** Healthy fats from sources like avocados, olive oil, and fatty fish can improve fat metabolism and prevent fatty liver disease.

How to Support Liver Health Through Diet:

- **Eat Whole, Plant-Based Foods:** Incorporate a variety of colorful fruits and vegetables, leafy greens, legumes, and whole grains into your daily meals to provide essential nutrients.
- **Healthy Fats:** Include healthy fats from sources like olive oil, nuts, seeds, and fatty fish (salmon, sardines) to support liver function and reduce liver fat.

- **Limit Sugar and Processed Foods:** Reduce consumption of refined sugars, processed meats, and fried foods that can overload the liver with toxins and promote fat accumulation.
- **Hydrating Foods:** Include water-rich foods such as cucumbers, watermelon, and celery in your diet to support hydration.

5. Manage Stress Effectively

Chronic stress can negatively affect liver function. When you experience stress, your body releases **cortisol**, a hormone that, in excess, can promote fat accumulation in the liver and contribute to inflammation. Moreover, stress can lead to unhealthy eating habits, such as consuming comfort foods or alcohol, which can further harm liver health.

Why Stress Management Supports Liver Health:

- **Reduces Inflammation:** Chronic stress increases inflammation in the body, which can negatively impact liver function. Managing stress helps lower cortisol levels, which can reduce inflammation.
- **Promotes Healthy Habits:** Stress management techniques, such as mindfulness, meditation, or exercise, encourage healthier choices, which ultimately benefit liver health.
- **Supports Digestive Health:** Stress can impact digestion, leading to poor nutrient absorption and additional strain on the liver. Stress reduction supports better digestion and nutrient assimilation.

How to Manage Stress:

- **Mindfulness & Meditation:** Practice mindfulness techniques, such as deep breathing exercises or guided meditation, to help calm your nervous system.
- **Physical Activity:** Engage in regular physical activity, which has been shown to reduce cortisol levels and improve mood.
- **Relaxation Techniques:** Explore relaxation practices such as progressive muscle relaxation, aromatherapy, or taking relaxing baths to alleviate tension.

6. Avoid Toxins and Harmful Substances

To protect the liver, it's important to avoid substances that can overwhelm or damage it. Common liver stressors include alcohol, smoking, environmental toxins, and overuse of medications, especially pain relievers like acetaminophen (Tylenol).

Why Avoiding Toxins is Essential for Liver Health:

- **Alcohol and Medications:** Chronic alcohol consumption and the overuse of medications can damage liver cells and lead to conditions such as alcoholic liver disease or non-alcoholic fatty liver disease.
- **Environmental Toxins:** Exposure to chemicals, such as pesticides, heavy metals, and industrial pollutants, can accumulate in the liver and impair its ability to detoxify effectively.

How to Limit Toxin Exposure:

- **Limit Alcohol Consumption:** If you drink alcohol, do so in moderation. Avoid binge drinking, which can overwhelm the liver and cause long-term damage.
- **Use Medications Wisely:** Follow the instructions for any over-the-counter or prescription medications and avoid long-term overuse. Consult a healthcare provider for alternatives when needed.
- **Minimize Exposure to Chemicals:** Avoid unnecessary exposure to household chemicals, pesticides, and other environmental toxins by using natural cleaning products and minimizing the use of chemical-based personal care items.

Chapter 7: Exercise for Liver Health – Best Practices for Fatty Liver Reversal

Exercise plays a pivotal role in maintaining liver health and is a key component in reversing fatty liver disease. Whether you're dealing with non-alcoholic fatty liver disease (NAFLD), alcohol-related liver damage, or any other liver dysfunction, regular physical activity can significantly improve liver function, reduce fat accumulation, and enhance overall metabolic health. In this chapter, we'll dive into the science behind how exercise benefits the liver and provide practical advice on the best types of exercise to promote fatty liver reversal.

Why Exercise is Crucial for Liver Health

The liver is responsible for several vital functions, including detoxification, nutrient metabolism, bile production, and fat storage. When the liver becomes overburdened with fat, it leads to fatty liver disease. Exercise can help reverse or prevent this condition in several key ways:

- **Improves Insulin Sensitivity:** Insulin resistance is a common precursor to fatty liver disease. Exercise helps reduce insulin resistance by increasing the muscle cells' sensitivity to insulin, improving glucose metabolism, and reducing excess fat in the liver.
- **Promotes Fat Loss:** Regular exercise increases energy expenditure, helping you lose excess body fat. Reducing fat accumulation, particularly around the abdomen, is critical for liver health. Abdominal fat (visceral fat) is strongly associated with non-alcoholic fatty liver disease (NAFLD) and other metabolic disorders.

- **Reduces Inflammation:** Chronic low-grade inflammation is a hallmark of fatty liver disease. Physical activity, particularly aerobic exercises, has anti-inflammatory effects and can help reduce liver inflammation.
- **Enhances Fat Oxidation:** Exercise, especially aerobic and resistance training, helps the liver metabolize fats more efficiently. This reduces fat accumulation and supports fat-burning processes in the liver.
- **Improves Blood Circulation:** Regular exercise improves overall blood circulation, which helps deliver oxygen and nutrients to liver cells and promotes detoxification.

By incorporating a structured exercise routine into your daily life, you can support liver detoxification, improve fat metabolism, and reduce liver fat. Let's explore the types of exercise that are particularly beneficial for fatty liver reversal.

Best Types of Exercise for Fatty Liver Disease Reversal

1. Aerobic Exercise (Cardio)

Aerobic exercises, or cardio, are one of the most effective forms of exercise for improving liver health. These activities increase heart rate and improve blood flow, promoting fat burning and enhancing liver detoxification.

How Aerobic Exercise Helps the Liver:

- **Fat Loss:** Cardio helps you burn calories and reduce body fat, which is essential for reversing fatty liver

disease. Studies show that regular aerobic activity can lead to a significant reduction in liver fat.
- **Improved Insulin Sensitivity:** Aerobic exercise improves insulin sensitivity, which reduces fat accumulation in the liver. This is crucial for reversing insulin resistance, which often accompanies fatty liver disease.
- **Increased Energy Expenditure:** Regular cardio helps increase energy expenditure, making it easier to maintain a healthy weight and prevent the progression of fatty liver.

Examples of Aerobic Exercise:

- **Walking:** A low-impact, easy-to-do activity that's great for beginners. Aim for 30–60 minutes of brisk walking, 5–7 days a week.
- **Jogging or Running:** More intense than walking, jogging and running can help you burn more calories and fat. Start slow and gradually increase duration and intensity.
- **Cycling:** Whether outdoors or on a stationary bike, cycling provides an excellent aerobic workout that can help with weight loss and improve cardiovascular health.
- **Swimming:** A full-body workout that is easy on the joints but effective in increasing heart rate and improving overall fat-burning capacity.
- **Dancing:** Dance-based fitness classes (e.g., Zumba, aerobics) are fun and engaging ways to get your heart rate up while enjoying the benefits of cardio exercise.

Recommended Duration & Frequency:

- **Moderate-intensity exercise:** Aim for at least 150 minutes per week (e.g., 30 minutes, 5 days a week).
- **High-intensity interval training (HIIT):** If you're more advanced, HIIT can be effective for fat burning. Incorporate it 2–3 times per week for 20–30 minutes.

2. Resistance Training (Strength Training)

While aerobic exercise is important for fat loss, resistance training (also known as strength training or weightlifting) plays a complementary role in reversing fatty liver disease. Strength training builds muscle mass, which in turn boosts metabolism and helps the body burn more fat, even at rest.

How Resistance Training Benefits the Liver:

- **Increases Muscle Mass:** The more muscle mass you have, the more calories you burn, even at rest. This helps with weight management, which is crucial for reversing fatty liver disease.
- **Enhances Insulin Sensitivity:** Strength training has been shown to improve insulin sensitivity, which reduces fat accumulation in the liver.
- **Improves Fat Metabolism:** Building muscle through resistance training can help the liver more effectively metabolize fat and improve liver function overall.

Examples of Resistance Training Exercises:

- **Bodyweight Exercises:** Push-ups, squats, lunges, and planks are all effective bodyweight exercises that target multiple muscle groups.

- **Free Weights:** Dumbbells, kettlebells, or barbells can be used to target specific muscle groups. Start with lighter weights and gradually increase the load as you build strength.
- **Resistance Bands:** Resistance bands are a low-impact, portable option that can be used to strengthen muscles without putting too much strain on the joints.
- **Machines:** If you have access to a gym, weight machines can be useful for targeting specific muscle groups, especially for beginners.

Recommended Duration & Frequency:

- Aim for **2–3 strength training sessions per week**.
- Include exercises that target all major muscle groups (legs, back, chest, arms, and core).

3. High-Intensity Interval Training (HIIT)

High-Intensity Interval Training (HIIT) combines short bursts of intense exercise followed by brief recovery periods. HIIT has gained popularity due to its effectiveness in burning fat, increasing muscle mass, and improving cardiovascular health, all of which can benefit the liver.

How HIIT Supports Fatty Liver Reversal:

- **Enhanced Fat Burning:** HIIT has been shown to be highly effective for burning fat, particularly visceral fat, which is directly linked to fatty liver disease.
- **Improved Metabolic Health:** HIIT improves insulin sensitivity, lowers blood sugar, and boosts fat oxidation, all of which are critical for reversing fatty liver disease.

- **Time-Efficient:** HIIT workouts can be completed in a short period, making them ideal for those with limited time.

Examples of HIIT Exercises:

- **Sprint Intervals:** Alternate between sprinting and walking for 20–30 minutes.
- **Jump Squats & Burpees:** Perform explosive movements like jump squats, burpees, and mountain climbers in short bursts followed by brief rest periods.
- **Circuit Training:** Combine strength exercises (e.g., push-ups, squats, lunges) with brief cardio bursts (e.g., jumping jacks or running in place).

Recommended Duration & Frequency:

- **20–30 minutes per session**, 2–3 times per week.
- Ensure at least one rest day between HIIT workouts to allow recovery.

4. Yoga and Stretching

While yoga and stretching exercises may not be as intense as aerobic or resistance training, they offer significant benefits for overall liver health. Yoga helps reduce stress, improve circulation, and support the body's natural detoxification processes.

How Yoga and Stretching Benefit Liver Health:

- **Stress Reduction:** Yoga activates the parasympathetic nervous system, reducing stress and cortisol levels, which can negatively affect liver health.
- **Improves Circulation:** Many yoga poses promote better blood circulation, which supports liver function and detoxification.
- **Detoxification:** Certain yoga poses, like twists and forward bends, are believed to stimulate liver function and aid in the detoxification process.
- **Enhances Flexibility:** Stretching helps improve flexibility and prevent muscle stiffness, which can lead to better posture and overall well-being.

Examples of Yoga Poses for Liver Health:

- **Twisted Chair Pose (Parivrtta Utkatasana):** This pose involves a seated twist that massages the liver and encourages detoxification.
- **Bridge Pose (Setu Bandhasana):** A backbend that opens up the chest and stimulates the digestive system, promoting liver detox.
- **Forward Fold (Uttanasana):** A standing forward bend that helps increase circulation to the liver and kidneys.

Recommended Duration & Frequency:

- Aim for **20–30 minutes of yoga** 2–3 times a week.
- Include gentle stretches daily to improve flexibility and circulation.

Exercise That Supports Liver Healing: The Role of Cardiovascular and Resistance Training in Reversing Fatty Liver

Fatty liver disease, particularly non-alcoholic fatty liver disease (NAFLD), is increasingly prevalent worldwide, often driven by poor diet, lack of exercise, and obesity. When excess fat accumulates in the liver cells, it can lead to inflammation, liver damage, and in severe cases, cirrhosis. While dietary changes are essential in addressing fatty liver, exercise plays a critical role in promoting liver health and reversing the condition. Specifically, cardiovascular (cardio) exercise and resistance training have been shown to provide substantial benefits in reducing liver fat, improving liver function, and supporting long-term liver healing.

In this article, we will explore the specific ways in which cardiovascular and resistance training contribute to liver healing, with a focus on how these types of exercise can help reverse fatty liver disease.

How Exercise Affects Fatty Liver Disease

The liver is responsible for a variety of essential functions, including detoxification, nutrient metabolism, and fat storage. When the liver becomes overloaded with fat, it can no longer perform these functions effectively. Fatty liver disease often accompanies obesity, insulin resistance, and metabolic syndrome, all of which increase the risk of liver damage. Exercise, especially when combined with dietary changes, can help reverse fatty liver by addressing the root causes of the disease:

- **Reduces Fat Accumulation in the Liver:** Exercise helps burn excess fat, particularly visceral fat (fat around the organs), which is closely linked to fatty liver disease.
- **Improves Insulin Sensitivity:** Insulin resistance, a hallmark of fatty liver disease, impairs the body's ability to process glucose and store fat properly. Exercise improves insulin sensitivity, allowing the body to regulate blood sugar and fat metabolism more efficiently.
- **Reduces Liver Inflammation:** Chronic inflammation is a key factor in the progression of fatty liver disease. Regular exercise has anti-inflammatory effects that help reduce liver inflammation and promote healing.
- **Enhances Liver Detoxification:** Physical activity supports the liver's natural detox processes by improving circulation, stimulating bile production, and aiding in the removal of waste products.

Now, let's dive deeper into how two primary forms of exercise—cardiovascular training and resistance training—can promote liver healing.

Cardiovascular Exercise: A Key to Fatty Liver Reversal

Cardiovascular exercise, often referred to as aerobic exercise, is one of the most effective forms of exercise for managing and reversing fatty liver disease. It includes activities that elevate your heart rate and improve cardiovascular health, such as walking, running, cycling, and swimming.

How Cardiovascular Exercise Supports Liver Healing:

1. **Fat Burning and Weight Loss:**
   - One of the primary ways cardio helps reverse fatty liver disease is through fat loss. Cardiovascular exercise increases the body's calorie expenditure, helping you burn stored fat, especially visceral fat. Reducing fat around the liver reduces liver fat content and prevents further liver damage.
   - A study published in *Hepatology* found that aerobic exercise could reduce liver fat in individuals with NAFLD, even without significant weight loss. The combination of fat-burning exercise and a reduced calorie diet can lead to substantial reductions in liver fat and overall body weight.
2. **Improved Insulin Sensitivity:**
   - Insulin resistance, which is often seen in individuals with fatty liver, impairs the liver's ability to metabolize fat and glucose. Cardio exercises improve insulin sensitivity by increasing glucose uptake in muscle cells and improving fat metabolism. This helps the liver burn fat more efficiently and reduces fat accumulation.
   - Research has shown that consistent aerobic exercise significantly improves insulin sensitivity, which can help reduce fat build-up in the liver and reduce the risk of progressing to more severe liver damage.
3. **Reduced Inflammation:**
   - Chronic inflammation is a major contributor to the development and progression of fatty liver disease. Regular cardio exercise has been shown

to have anti-inflammatory effects, helping to reduce liver inflammation and preventing liver fibrosis (scarring).
- A study published in *The Journal of Clinical Endocrinology & Metabolism* found that aerobic exercise reduced markers of inflammation in people with fatty liver disease, supporting the healing process and reducing the likelihood of liver damage.

4. **Enhanced Circulation and Detoxification:**
   - Cardio exercise improves blood circulation, which helps deliver oxygen and nutrients to the liver cells. Enhanced circulation also facilitates the removal of toxins and metabolic waste from the liver, aiding in detoxification.
   - Better circulation encourages the liver to function optimally, boosting its detoxification processes and supporting overall liver health.

Examples of Cardiovascular Exercises:

- **Walking:** Low-impact, easy to do, and effective for beginners. Aim for brisk walking for 30–60 minutes, 5–7 days a week.
- **Running or Jogging:** A higher-intensity form of cardio that helps burn fat faster. Start slow and build up to longer sessions.
- **Cycling:** Whether on a stationary bike or outdoors, cycling is an excellent way to get your heart rate up and burn fat.
- **Swimming:** A full-body, low-impact workout that's easy on the joints but effective at burning fat.

- **HIIT (High-Intensity Interval Training):** Short bursts of high-intensity exercise followed by brief rest periods. HIIT has been shown to be highly effective at reducing visceral fat and improving liver function.

Resistance Training: Building Muscle to Improve Liver Health

While cardiovascular exercise is effective for fat loss, resistance training (strength training) plays an equally important role in supporting liver healing. Resistance training involves exercises that target specific muscle groups using weights, resistance bands, or bodyweight exercises.

How Resistance Training Helps Reverse Fatty Liver Disease:

1. **Increased Muscle Mass and Metabolic Rate:**
    - Building muscle through resistance training boosts your metabolism by increasing the number of calories you burn, even at rest. Muscle tissue burns more calories than fat tissue, making it easier to maintain a healthy weight and prevent fat accumulation in the liver.
    - Increased muscle mass helps reduce fat, including liver fat, by improving overall fat metabolism and promoting fat oxidation. As muscle mass increases, the liver is less likely to accumulate fat.
2. **Improved Insulin Sensitivity and Blood Sugar Regulation:**

- Just like cardio, resistance training enhances insulin sensitivity. Strength training increases glucose uptake by muscle cells, helping the body regulate blood sugar levels more effectively and reducing the load on the liver.
- A study published in *The Journal of Strength and Conditioning Research* found that strength training improved insulin sensitivity in individuals with NAFLD, making it easier for the liver to process and store nutrients.

3. **Reduction in Visceral Fat:**
   - Resistance training helps reduce visceral fat (fat around the organs), which is strongly associated with fatty liver disease. By targeting this fat, resistance training reduces liver fat and promotes liver healing.
   - Resistance training combined with aerobic exercise has been shown to result in significant reductions in visceral fat, providing a dual benefit for fatty liver disease reversal.

4. **Support for Overall Health:**
   - Strength training not only benefits the liver but also supports overall physical health. Improved muscle strength, bone density, and cardiovascular function all contribute to a healthier body, which in turn benefits the liver.

Examples of Resistance Training Exercises:

- **Bodyweight Exercises:** Squats, push-ups, lunges, and planks are great starting points for building strength without any equipment.

- **Free Weights:** Dumbbells, kettlebells, or barbells can be used for exercises like deadlifts, bench presses, and rows to target different muscle groups.
- **Resistance Bands:** A portable, low-impact option for strengthening muscles and improving flexibility.
- **Machines:** Weight machines can also be used for specific muscle groups, especially for beginners.

Recommended Frequency and Duration:

- **Strength training 2-3 times per week.**
- **Aim for 30–45 minutes per session,** focusing on major muscle groups like legs, back, chest, arms, and core.

The Perfect Combination: Cardiovascular and Resistance Training for Liver Health

To maximize the benefits for fatty liver reversal, it's essential to combine both cardiovascular and resistance training into a well-rounded exercise routine. Cardiovascular exercise helps burn fat and improves insulin sensitivity, while resistance training builds muscle mass, enhances metabolism, and reduces visceral fat.

A balanced exercise program might look like this:

- **Cardio:** 3–5 days per week, 30–60 minutes per session (moderate to intense).
- **Strength Training:** 2–3 days per week, 30–45 minutes per session, targeting all major muscle groups.

This combination not only helps reverse fatty liver disease but also improves overall metabolic health, reduces the risk of cardiovascular disease, and promotes weight management, which is essential for maintaining liver health.

Understanding Fat-Burning Workouts: Why Fat-Burning Exercises Are Key for Fatty Liver Disease Management

Fatty liver disease, particularly non-alcoholic fatty liver disease (NAFLD), is a growing health concern that affects millions of people worldwide. It is characterized by the accumulation of fat in liver cells, which can lead to inflammation, scarring, and even cirrhosis if left untreated. One of the most effective ways to manage and even reverse fatty liver disease is through fat-burning exercises. These exercises not only help reduce the amount of fat stored in the liver but also improve overall metabolic health, which is essential for liver function.

In this article, we will explore why fat-burning exercises are crucial for managing fatty liver disease, how they work, and the best types of workouts to support liver health.

How Fat-Burning Exercises Support Fatty Liver Disease Management

Fatty liver disease is often associated with metabolic disorders such as obesity, insulin resistance, and high cholesterol. The liver plays a critical role in metabolizing fats and detoxifying the body, but when it becomes overloaded with fat, it can no longer perform these functions effectively. This can lead to a vicious cycle of fat accumulation, liver dysfunction, and inflammation. Fat-burning exercises can help break this cycle by promoting fat loss, improving insulin sensitivity, and reducing liver inflammation.

Here's how fat-burning exercises support fatty liver disease management:

1. **Reduction of Liver Fat:**
   - The primary goal in managing fatty liver disease is to reduce the amount of fat in the liver. Fat-burning exercises, especially those that increase your heart rate and promote calorie expenditure, help burn stored fat throughout the body, including in the liver. By reducing fat accumulation in the liver, fat-burning workouts can prevent or even reverse liver damage caused by excess fat.
2. **Improvement in Insulin Sensitivity:**
   - Insulin resistance is a common condition in individuals with fatty liver disease. It occurs when the body's cells become less responsive to insulin, leading to higher blood sugar levels and increased fat storage, including in the liver. Fat-burning exercises improve insulin sensitivity by allowing the body's cells to more efficiently process glucose and store fat. As a result, regular fat-burning workouts help lower the risk of developing diabetes and improve fat metabolism, reducing fat buildup in the liver.
3. **Increased Calorie Expenditure and Weight Loss:**
   - Fat-burning exercises increase the body's calorie expenditure, which helps create a calorie

deficit—an essential component of weight loss. Losing weight is one of the most effective ways to reduce liver fat. Even modest weight loss (5-10% of body weight) can significantly improve liver function and reduce fat buildup in the liver. Fat-burning workouts, when combined with a healthy diet, support weight loss and promote a healthier liver.

4. **Reduction of Visceral Fat:**
   - Visceral fat, the fat that accumulates around internal organs such as the liver, is strongly linked to fatty liver disease. Fat-burning exercises, especially those that involve whole-body movements, help target visceral fat. By reducing visceral fat, these exercises help decrease liver fat, improve liver function, and reduce the risk of complications associated with fatty liver disease, such as liver fibrosis or cirrhosis.

5. **Reduction of Inflammation:**
   - Chronic low-grade inflammation is a hallmark of fatty liver disease and contributes to liver damage and fibrosis. Regular fat-burning exercise has been shown to have anti-inflammatory effects, helping to reduce liver inflammation and promote healing. This can be particularly beneficial for individuals with non-alcoholic steatohepatitis (NASH), a more severe form of fatty liver disease that involves inflammation and liver cell injury.

Types of Fat-Burning Workouts for Fatty Liver Disease

There are various types of fat-burning exercises, each with its own benefits. The most effective fat-burning workouts combine both cardiovascular (aerobic) exercise and resistance (strength) training. Here's a breakdown of the best types of fat-burning exercises to include in a liver-healthy routine:

1. Cardiovascular (Aerobic) Exercises: The Heart of Fat Burning

Cardiovascular exercises, also known as aerobic exercises, are the most effective way to burn calories and fat. These exercises increase your heart rate, improve circulation, and elevate calorie burn, which directly contributes to fat loss. When done regularly, cardiovascular exercise helps reduce the fat stored in the liver, improve insulin sensitivity, and boost liver function.

Types of Cardiovascular Exercises:

- **Walking or Brisk Walking:** A low-impact exercise that's easy on the joints and can be done daily. Aim for 30-60 minutes per day to burn fat and improve liver health.
- **Running or Jogging:** Higher intensity than walking, running helps burn more calories and is excellent for fat loss. Start slow and gradually increase distance and speed.

- **Cycling:** Both outdoor cycling and stationary cycling are effective for burning fat. Cycling engages the lower body muscles and helps improve cardiovascular health.
- **Swimming:** A full-body workout that's easy on the joints while providing an excellent cardiovascular workout. Swimming can be particularly beneficial for people with joint issues or those who are overweight.
- **High-Intensity Interval Training (HIIT):** Short bursts of intense activity followed by periods of rest. HIIT is highly effective for burning fat quickly and improving cardiovascular fitness. Studies show that HIIT can be more effective than steady-state cardio in reducing liver fat and improving metabolic health.

Benefits of Cardiovascular Exercises for Fatty Liver Disease:

- **Fat loss:** Helps burn both visceral and liver fat.
- **Improved insulin sensitivity:** Reduces the risk of type 2 diabetes.
- **Increased energy:** Boosts overall vitality and stamina.
- **Heart health:** Improves cardiovascular function and reduces the risk of heart disease, which is common among individuals with fatty liver disease.

2. Resistance Training: Building Muscle to Burn More Fat

While cardiovascular exercises are great for burning calories and improving cardiovascular health, resistance training is essential for building muscle mass and boosting metabolism. Muscle tissue burns more calories at rest than fat tissue, so increasing muscle mass can help you burn more fat, even when you're not exercising. Resistance training also targets visceral fat and supports overall metabolic health.

Types of Resistance Training Exercises:

- **Bodyweight Exercises:** Squats, lunges, push-ups, and planks are excellent starting points for building strength without any equipment. These exercises engage multiple muscle groups, helping to increase muscle mass and burn fat.
- **Dumbbells or Free Weights:** Incorporating free weights into your routine (e.g., bicep curls, shoulder presses, deadlifts) helps build muscle and increase overall calorie burn.
- **Resistance Bands:** These are affordable, portable tools that can provide resistance for exercises like squats, leg presses, and arm exercises.
- **Weight Machines:** If you have access to a gym, machines can help target specific muscle groups, especially for beginners.

Benefits of Resistance Training for Fatty Liver Disease:

- **Muscle building:** Increases lean muscle mass, which boosts metabolism and helps with fat loss.
- **Improved fat metabolism:** Resistance training helps regulate blood sugar and promotes fat-burning.
- **Enhanced insulin sensitivity:** Like cardio, resistance training improves insulin sensitivity, which is crucial for managing fatty liver disease.
- **Reduced visceral fat:** Targets abdominal and visceral fat, which is directly linked to fatty liver.

3. Combining Cardio and Strength Training for Optimal Fat Burning

The most effective approach for burning fat and reversing fatty liver disease is to combine cardiovascular exercise with resistance training. This combination maximizes fat loss, improves insulin sensitivity, and helps maintain lean muscle mass while reducing liver fat.

Sample Weekly Routine for Fat-Burning and Liver Health:

- **3 days of cardio:** 30-60 minutes of moderate to intense aerobic exercise (e.g., brisk walking, cycling, or HIIT).
- **2-3 days of strength training:** 30-45 minutes of resistance exercises (e.g., bodyweight exercises, free weights, or resistance bands).
- **1-2 days of active rest:** Engage in light activities like walking or stretching to keep the body moving without overexertion.

How to Create a Sustainable Exercise Routine: Tips for Integrating Exercise into Daily Life Without Overwhelming Yourself

Creating a sustainable exercise routine is essential for long-term health and wellness. But with busy schedules, stress, and the constant demands of life, finding a way to incorporate regular physical activity can feel daunting. The key is to build a routine that is realistic, flexible, and enjoyable so that it becomes a natural part of your daily life rather than something you dread or feel overwhelmed by.

In this guide, we will explore practical tips and strategies for creating a sustainable exercise routine that fits seamlessly into your life while helping you achieve your fitness and health goals.

1. Start Small and Gradually Build Up

The most important rule when starting a new exercise routine is to avoid jumping in too quickly. Trying to do too much at once can lead to burnout, injury, or frustration. Instead, begin with small, manageable goals and gradually increase your workout intensity, duration, or frequency over time. This approach allows your body to adjust and builds momentum without overwhelming you.

Tips for Getting Started:

- **Set Realistic Goals:** Aim for 10-15 minutes of exercise per day at the beginning, and increase it by 5-10 minutes each week as your fitness improves.
- **Focus on Consistency, Not Intensity:** It's more important to make exercise a regular habit than to push yourself too hard in the beginning. A consistent, low-intensity routine is better for long-term success than sporadic, intense workouts.
- **Track Your Progress:** Use a journal or fitness app to track your workouts. Seeing your improvement over time is motivating and helps you stay on track.

2. Find Activities You Enjoy

One of the biggest reasons people fall off their exercise routines is that they engage in activities they don't enjoy. If exercise feels like a chore, it's easy to put it off or abandon it entirely. The key to sustainability is finding physical activities that bring you joy. When you enjoy what you're doing, it doesn't feel like work, and you're more likely to stick with it.

Ideas for Fun and Engaging Exercises:

- **Dance:** Whether it's hip-hop, salsa, or just dancing to your favorite songs at home, dance is a great way to get moving and have fun.
- **Walking or Hiking:** Walking is a low-impact and easy activity that you can do anywhere. Explore nature trails or take a walk around your neighborhood.
- **Swimming:** Swimming is gentle on the joints and provides a full-body workout, making it ideal for people of all fitness levels.
- **Cycling:** Whether outdoors or on a stationary bike, cycling is a fun way to get your heart pumping while enjoying the scenery.
- **Group Classes:** If you enjoy social interaction, try group fitness classes like yoga, pilates, spin, or Zumba. The energy of a group can keep you motivated.

3. Make It a Part of Your Daily Routine

To make exercise sustainable, it's crucial to incorporate it into your daily routine. This helps establish it as a non-negotiable habit, just like eating, sleeping, or brushing your teeth.

Creating a routine that fits into your day's rhythm will make it easier to stick to over time.

How to Integrate Exercise Into Your Routine:

- **Schedule It:** Treat your workout like any other important appointment. Put it on your calendar and set reminders to ensure you don't forget or skip it.
- **Exercise in the Morning:** Morning workouts are a great way to set the tone for your day. By getting your exercise done early, you won't be as likely to skip it due to work, fatigue, or distractions later in the day.
- **Break It Into Short Sessions:** If a long workout doesn't fit into your day, break it into shorter sessions. For example, do a 10-minute workout in the morning, another during lunch, and a third in the evening. These short bursts of activity can still have significant benefits and won't feel overwhelming.
- **Combine Activities:** Look for opportunities to combine exercise with other daily tasks. Walk or bike to work, take the stairs instead of the elevator, or do a quick workout while watching TV.

4. Mix Up Your Routine to Keep It Fresh

Repetition can lead to boredom, which can make it harder to stay committed to your exercise routine. To avoid this, make sure to mix up your activities. Not only will this keep things interesting, but it will also engage different muscle groups, reduce the risk of overuse injuries, and help you see better results.

How to Keep Your Routine Fresh:

- **Alternate Between Cardio and Strength Training:** For example, one day you might go for a jog or do a cycling class, and the next day you might focus on resistance training with weights or bodyweight exercises.
- **Try New Classes or Workouts:** Explore different types of workouts that are available to you, like yoga, pilates, barre, or martial arts. If you're exercising at home, try following a new workout video on YouTube or an app.
- **Seasonal Activities:** Engage in activities that are specific to the season. For example, you can enjoy outdoor activities like hiking, biking, or swimming during warmer months, and transition to indoor exercises like yoga or weightlifting during colder months.

5. Focus on Recovery and Listen to Your Body

A sustainable exercise routine isn't just about working hard; it's about working smart. Recovery is essential for long-term success. Overtraining can lead to burnout, injury, and fatigue, making it harder to stay consistent. Listening to your body and giving it time to recover ensures that you can continue exercising without feeling drained.

Recovery Tips:

- **Rest Days:** Incorporate rest days into your weekly routine. Rest allows your muscles to repair and grow, helping you avoid fatigue and injuries.

- **Sleep:** Aim for 7-9 hours of quality sleep each night. Sleep is essential for muscle recovery and overall well-being.
- **Stretching and Foam Rolling:** After your workouts, spend some time stretching and using a foam roller to release tension and improve flexibility. This will help prevent injuries and reduce soreness.
- **Stay Hydrated:** Drink plenty of water throughout the day to keep your body hydrated, especially during and after exercise. Proper hydration supports muscle function and recovery.

6. Build a Support System for Accountability

Having a support system can make all the difference when it comes to sticking with your exercise routine. Whether it's a friend, family member, workout buddy, or an online community, accountability will keep you motivated and make exercising more enjoyable.

Ways to Stay Accountable:

- **Join a Group or Class:** Participating in group fitness classes or online workout communities provides support and motivation from others.
- **Find a Workout Buddy:** Partner up with a friend or family member who shares similar fitness goals. Having someone to exercise with can make the experience more fun and help you stay committed.
- **Use Fitness Apps or Trackers:** Many fitness apps and wearables can help you track your progress, set goals, and receive reminders to stay active.

7. Celebrate Your Successes and Adjust as Needed

Sustainability also comes from celebrating your progress, no matter how small. Recognizing the improvements you've made will help you stay motivated and committed to your exercise routine. It's also important to remain flexible and adjust your routine when necessary. Life changes, and so do your fitness needs.

How to Celebrate Your Successes:

- **Track Milestones:** Keep a journal of your progress—whether it's in terms of strength, endurance, weight loss, or consistency. Celebrate when you hit milestones like completing your first 30-minute workout or reaching a weekly exercise goal.
- **Reward Yourself:** Reward yourself for sticking to your routine. This could be as simple as a relaxing bath after a workout, a new pair of workout clothes, or a fun activity you enjoy.
- **Reassess Your Routine:** If your routine stops feeling sustainable or enjoyable, reassess it. Make changes based on what's working and what isn't.

Chapter 8: Managing Stress and Emotional Health – A Key Component in Reversing Fatty Liver

The health of our liver is intricately tied to our overall well-being, and one of the most overlooked factors in liver health is the role that stress and emotional health play. Chronic stress, emotional instability, and negative mental states can significantly impact the body's ability to heal, including the reversal of fatty liver disease. In this chapter, we will explore the connection between stress, emotional health, and fatty liver disease, and offer practical strategies to manage stress effectively, promote emotional well-being, and support the liver's healing process.

The Link Between Stress, Emotional Health, and Fatty Liver Disease

Understanding how stress affects liver health is crucial in managing fatty liver disease (FLD). When we experience stress, whether physical, emotional, or mental, our bodies initiate the "fight or flight" response, which releases stress hormones such as cortisol and adrenaline. While these hormones are helpful in short bursts (for example, when we're in danger), chronic stress leads to prolonged elevations in these hormones, which can have damaging effects on the liver and overall health.

Here's how stress can specifically impact liver health:

1. **Increased Inflammation:** Chronic stress contributes to systemic inflammation, a key factor in the development and progression of fatty liver disease. Inflammation can

lead to oxidative stress, which damages liver cells and hinders their ability to regenerate.
2. **Insulin Resistance:** Stress hormones interfere with insulin sensitivity, contributing to insulin resistance. This condition is commonly seen in fatty liver disease and is a precursor to Type 2 diabetes. Insulin resistance reduces the liver's ability to metabolize fats efficiently, leading to fat accumulation in liver cells.
3. **Fat Accumulation:** Stress can increase fat storage in the liver. Elevated cortisol levels promote the storage of visceral fat (fat around internal organs), including the liver, which contributes to fatty liver disease.
4. **Disruption of Healthy Eating Patterns:** Chronic stress often leads to poor eating habits. Many individuals turn to unhealthy comfort foods, which are typically high in sugar, fat, and processed carbohydrates. These foods contribute to weight gain and further exacerbate liver health issues.
5. **Liver Detoxification Impairment:** Stress can impair the liver's ability to detoxify the body. Under stress, the liver's metabolic processes become sluggish, making it harder to eliminate toxins, heavy metals, and metabolic by-products, which can accumulate and further stress the liver.

The Role of Emotional Health in Fatty Liver Reversal

Emotional health and mental well-being play a key role in liver healing and disease management. Emotional distress, such as anxiety, depression, and unresolved trauma, can create a biochemical imbalance in the body, triggering physical changes that impact the liver. Here's how emotional health affects liver function:

1. **Psychological Stress and the Liver:** Chronic emotional stress, such as anxiety or depression, can lead to constant activation of the sympathetic nervous system, which can impair liver function over time. This results in reduced liver detoxification capacity, disrupted hormone balance, and a weakened immune system.
2. **Gut-Liver Connection:** Emotions also affect the gut-brain axis, the bidirectional communication between the brain and gut. Emotional distress can lead to gut dysbiosis (an imbalance in gut bacteria), which can exacerbate liver inflammation and contribute to the development of fatty liver disease. The gut and liver are closely connected, and an unhealthy gut can impair liver function.
3. **Cortisol and Liver Fat Storage:** Emotional stress triggers the release of cortisol, the body's primary stress hormone. Elevated cortisol not only causes fat to accumulate around internal organs (including the liver) but also promotes unhealthy eating patterns driven by emotional states. This results in weight gain and further liver stress.

Strategies for Managing Stress and Improving Emotional Health

To effectively reverse fatty liver disease, it's essential to adopt a holistic approach that includes stress management and emotional well-being. Below are evidence-based strategies to reduce stress, improve mental health, and promote liver healing:

1. Practice Mindfulness and Meditation

Mindfulness meditation is one of the most effective ways to reduce stress. Mindfulness involves focusing on the present moment without judgment, which helps you become aware of your thoughts and emotions without becoming overwhelmed by them. Regular mindfulness practice has been shown to reduce cortisol levels, lower inflammation, and improve emotional well-being.

How to Get Started:

- **Start Small:** Begin with 5-10 minutes of meditation each day, focusing on your breath and letting go of distracting thoughts.
- **Guided Meditation:** Use apps like Headspace, Calm, or Insight Timer for guided sessions that help you relax and center your mind.
- **Body Scan Meditation:** This practice involves focusing attention on different parts of your body, releasing tension, and promoting relaxation.

2. Exercise to Relieve Stress and Improve Mood

Regular physical activity is one of the best ways to manage stress. Exercise stimulates the release of endorphins, the body's natural mood enhancers. Cardiovascular exercises, in particular, improve blood flow and reduce cortisol levels, which supports liver function.

Recommended Exercises for Stress Relief:

- **Aerobic Exercise:** Walking, running, cycling, or swimming can help lower stress and improve overall fitness.
- **Strength Training:** Resistance training with weights or bodyweight exercises promotes muscle growth and helps regulate blood sugar levels, which is important for liver health.
- **Yoga and Pilates:** These mind-body practices combine physical movement with controlled breathing to reduce stress and improve flexibility.

3. Get Enough Restful Sleep

Sleep plays a crucial role in emotional regulation and overall health. Chronic stress and lack of sleep can disrupt hormone balance, including cortisol, and hinder the liver's ability to detoxify. Aim for 7-9 hours of sleep each night to give your body the time it needs to repair and rejuvenate, including liver regeneration.

Sleep Tips for Stress Management:

- **Establish a Sleep Routine:** Go to bed and wake up at the same time each day, even on weekends, to regulate your body's internal clock.
- **Create a Relaxing Sleep Environment:** Keep your bedroom cool, dark, and quiet. Avoid electronics at least an hour before bed to promote relaxation.
- **Use Relaxation Techniques:** Deep breathing, progressive muscle relaxation, or reading a calming

book before bed can help you unwind and prepare for sleep.

4. Cognitive Behavioral Therapy (CBT) and Counseling

For individuals dealing with anxiety, depression, or other emotional challenges, cognitive-behavioral therapy (CBT) can be an effective way to manage stress. CBT helps you identify and change negative thought patterns and behaviors that contribute to emotional distress. Counseling or therapy provides a safe space to process emotions and develop coping strategies.

Why CBT Helps:

- **Stress Management:** CBT helps identify triggers of emotional stress and equips individuals with tools to manage stress in a healthier way.
- **Addressing Negative Thought Patterns:** Therapy can help individuals change distorted thoughts that fuel anxiety and depression, leading to improved emotional health and reduced liver stress.

5. Practice Deep Breathing and Relaxation Techniques

Deep breathing exercises are simple yet powerful techniques to reduce the physical effects of stress on the body. Deep breathing helps lower heart rate, reduce blood pressure, and promote relaxation, all of which are beneficial for liver health.

Deep Breathing Exercises to Try:

- **Box Breathing:** Inhale for 4 counts, hold for 4 counts, exhale for 4 counts, and hold for 4 counts. Repeat this cycle for several minutes.
- **Diaphragmatic Breathing:** Focus on breathing deeply into your abdomen, not just your chest. This can help activate the parasympathetic nervous system, promoting relaxation.

6. Social Support and Connection

Human connection plays a critical role in managing stress and maintaining emotional health. Surrounding yourself with supportive friends, family members, or a community group provides a sense of belonging and emotional security. Studies show that social support helps reduce the physical effects of stress on the body, including inflammation and liver damage.

Ways to Foster Social Connection:

- **Join a Support Group:** Look for local or online groups focused on fatty liver disease or general wellness where you can share experiences and get advice.
- **Regular Social Interaction:** Make time for social activities that you enjoy, whether it's a hobby, a meetup, or spending quality time with loved ones.

7. Healthy Nutrition to Support Emotional Health

The foods we eat not only affect our liver but also play a critical role in mental health. Nutrient-dense foods, particularly those rich in omega-3 fatty acids, B-vitamins, antioxidants, and magnesium, can help balance brain chemistry, reduce stress, and improve emotional well-being.

Liver-Friendly Foods for Emotional Health:

- **Omega-3 Fatty Acids:** Found in fatty fish (salmon, mackerel), flaxseeds, and walnuts, omega-3s help reduce inflammation and support brain function.
- **Leafy Greens and Vegetables:** Rich in antioxidants and vitamins, these help combat oxidative stress and support the body's natural detoxification processes.
- **Complex Carbohydrates:** Whole grains, legumes, and vegetables provide a steady supply of energy, supporting stable blood sugar levels and mood regulation.

The Link Between Stress and Fatty Liver Disease

Fatty liver disease (FLD) is a growing health concern, often linked to poor dietary habits, obesity, and excessive alcohol consumption. However, one of the less-discussed factors that can have a profound impact on liver health is stress. While we typically associate stress with its mental and emotional effects, the way it influences the liver—especially in the context of fatty liver disease—deserves more attention. In this section, we will explore the connection between stress and fatty liver disease, focusing on how stress triggers hormonal imbalances, particularly elevated cortisol levels, which contribute to liver dysfunction.

How Stress Affects the Liver: A Biological Overview

The liver plays a central role in the body's detoxification processes, metabolism, and regulation of blood sugar. However, stress can significantly disrupt these processes. When the body experiences stress—whether it's emotional, mental, or physical—it activates the **hypothalamic-pituitary-adrenal (HPA) axis**. This is a complex system that governs the release of stress hormones, the most prominent of which is **cortisol**.

Cortisol, often referred to as the "stress hormone," is released by the adrenal glands in response to perceived threats. Under normal circumstances, cortisol is helpful in managing acute stress, increasing alertness, and providing the body with a burst of energy. However, chronic stress results in **prolonged elevated cortisol levels**, which have a cascade of detrimental effects on various body systems, including the liver.

The Role of Cortisol in Fatty Liver Disease

Cortisol's primary function is to regulate the body's stress response, but when chronically elevated, it can cause a series of metabolic disturbances that contribute to the development and progression of fatty liver disease. Here's how cortisol disrupts liver function:

1. Increased Fat Storage and Insulin Resistance

One of cortisol's primary effects on the body is its ability to influence fat storage. During periods of stress, cortisol directs the body to store fat, particularly in the abdominal area. This visceral fat is the type that accumulates around internal organs, including the liver.

When excess fat accumulates in liver cells, it leads to **non-alcoholic fatty liver disease (NAFLD)**. Additionally, prolonged exposure to high cortisol levels is linked to **insulin resistance**, a condition where the body's cells become less responsive to insulin. Insulin resistance prevents the liver from processing and storing glucose efficiently, leading to further fat buildup in liver cells.

2. Increased Inflammation and Oxidative Stress

Elevated cortisol levels are associated with increased inflammation in the body. In the context of the liver, this chronic inflammation contributes to **oxidative stress**, which is the damage caused by free radicals (unstable molecules) to liver cells.

Oxidative stress is a major contributor to liver damage and fibrosis, the process by which liver tissue becomes scarred. Chronic stress and the associated high cortisol levels not only promote fat storage but also fuel liver inflammation, which accelerates the progression from simple fatty liver to more severe conditions like **non-alcoholic steatohepatitis (NASH)** or **cirrhosis**.

3. Disruption of Liver Detoxification

The liver's primary function is detoxification—processing toxins and harmful substances that enter the body. When cortisol is elevated over long periods, the liver's ability to perform this crucial function can be compromised. Chronic stress can impair liver detoxification pathways, making it harder for the liver to process and eliminate toxins, including **toxins from food, alcohol, environmental pollutants**, and **metabolic waste products**.

As a result, these toxins accumulate in the body, leading to further stress on the liver and contributing to the development of liver disease. In the long run, this impaired detoxification can result in liver dysfunction and a diminished ability to repair itself.

Other Hormonal and Metabolic Changes Caused by Stress

Beyond cortisol, stress impacts several other hormones and metabolic processes that contribute to the development of fatty liver disease:

1. Disruption of Leptin and Ghrelin Levels

Leptin and ghrelin are hormones involved in regulating hunger and satiety. Leptin helps signal the brain when we are full, while ghrelin stimulates hunger. Stress can disrupt the balance of these hormones, leading to an increase in hunger and overeating. In particular, **stress-induced overconsumption of food** often involves unhealthy, calorie-dense, high-fat foods, which contribute to fat accumulation in the liver.

Furthermore, stress-induced overeating can cause fluctuations in blood sugar and insulin levels, exacerbating insulin resistance and further promoting fatty liver disease.

2. Alteration of Thyroid Function

The thyroid plays a vital role in regulating metabolism, including fat storage. Chronic stress can lead to **hypothyroidism** (underactive thyroid), where the thyroid doesn't produce enough hormones. When thyroid hormones are insufficient, metabolic processes slow down, and fat accumulates in the liver.

The imbalance between thyroid hormones and cortisol is particularly problematic because while cortisol encourages fat storage, a slow metabolism (due to hypothyroidism) prevents the body from effectively burning that fat. This contributes to the accumulation of fat in liver cells and the development of fatty liver disease.

3. Elevated Blood Pressure and Cardiovascular Strain

Chronic stress leads to increased blood pressure, which can further exacerbate liver health problems. High blood pressure is a known risk factor for **cardiovascular disease** and **fatty liver disease**. The cardiovascular strain caused by chronic stress can affect blood flow to the liver, impairing its ability to function optimally and increasing the risk of liver damage.

How Stress Management Can Help Reverse Fatty Liver Disease

Given the profound effects stress has on the liver, particularly in the context of fatty liver disease, managing stress is an essential part of any effective treatment or prevention strategy. Here are several methods that can help manage stress and support liver health:

1. Mindfulness and Meditation

Mindfulness practices, such as meditation, deep breathing, and body scans, have been shown to reduce cortisol levels and promote relaxation. By incorporating mindfulness into your daily routine, you can lower your stress levels and improve liver function by reducing the inflammatory effects of chronic stress.

2. Regular Exercise

Physical activity is a powerful tool for managing stress. Cardiovascular exercise, in particular, can help reduce cortisol levels, improve insulin sensitivity, and burn fat. Resistance training is also beneficial for increasing muscle mass, which helps regulate metabolism and improve liver health.

3. Healthy Diet and Nutrition

Maintaining a liver-friendly diet rich in antioxidants, healthy fats, and high-fiber foods can help reduce inflammation and oxidative stress caused by chronic cortisol elevation. Nutrients such as omega-3 fatty acids (found in fatty fish and flaxseeds) and antioxidants (found in fruits and vegetables) can support liver detoxification and healing.

4. Quality Sleep

Sleep is one of the most effective ways to regulate stress hormones. Poor sleep can lead to elevated cortisol levels, further exacerbating the effects of stress on the liver. Aim for 7-9 hours of restful sleep each night to help balance cortisol levels and support liver regeneration.

5. Social Support and Therapy

Having a strong social support network and engaging in counseling or therapy can significantly reduce emotional stress. Whether through talking to loved ones or seeking professional help, addressing emotional challenges can help lower cortisol levels and improve overall well-being.

Mindfulness, Meditation, and Relaxation Techniques: Simple Strategies to Reduce Stress and Support Overall Health

In today's fast-paced world, stress has become an almost constant companion for many people. From work pressures to personal challenges, stress can take a significant toll on both mental and physical health. Fortunately, mindfulness, meditation, and relaxation techniques offer a powerful and accessible way to reduce stress and support overall well-being. These practices have been proven to help manage emotional responses, regulate the nervous system, and promote a state of calm that benefits not just the mind, but the body as well.

In this section, we will explore the science behind mindfulness and meditation, their benefits for mental health, and simple techniques that can be easily integrated into your daily routine to reduce stress and improve overall health.

Understanding Mindfulness and Meditation

Mindfulness is the practice of being present in the moment, paying attention to your thoughts, feelings, and sensations without judgment. It's about noticing what's happening right now, rather than dwelling on the past or worrying about the future. Mindfulness can be cultivated through formal meditation practices or simply by becoming more aware of the present moment in everyday activities.

Meditation is a technique that helps enhance mindfulness. It often involves focusing on the breath, a mantra, or an image to quiet the mind and achieve a state of deep relaxation and heightened awareness. While mindfulness can be practiced at any moment of the day, meditation typically requires dedicated time to focus and engage with the practice more deeply.

Both mindfulness and meditation have been linked to numerous health benefits, including **stress reduction**, **improved emotional regulation**, **enhanced cognitive function**, **better sleep**, and even **reduced inflammation**.

The Science Behind Mindfulness and Meditation

Studies have shown that mindfulness and meditation have a profound impact on the brain and body. The **prefrontal cortex**, responsible for executive functions like decision-making, attention, and self-control, becomes more active during mindfulness practices. At the same time, mindfulness can reduce activity in the **amygdala**, the brain region associated with stress and emotional reactivity.

Additionally, research shows that regular mindfulness meditation can lower the levels of the **stress hormone cortisol**, reduce **blood pressure**, and promote a sense of overall well-being. These benefits contribute to improved mental clarity, emotional resilience, and better physical health.

Benefits of Mindfulness, Meditation, and Relaxation Techniques for Stress Reduction and Overall Health

1. **Reduction of Stress and Anxiety**
   Mindfulness practices have been shown to significantly reduce the symptoms of stress and anxiety. By focusing on the present moment, individuals are less likely to ruminate on past experiences or worry about the future—two common triggers of anxiety. Meditation, in particular, has been found to reduce **anxiety disorders**, including generalized anxiety disorder (GAD), by calming the nervous system and improving emotional regulation.
2. **Improved Emotional Regulation**
   Mindfulness and meditation help develop greater emotional awareness, allowing individuals to respond more thoughtfully to difficult situations. Instead of reacting impulsively to stressors, mindful practices encourage a more balanced approach to emotional challenges, promoting emotional resilience and self-compassion.
3. **Enhanced Sleep Quality**
   Stress is one of the most common causes of insomnia and poor sleep quality. Meditation techniques, such as deep breathing exercises or body scans, promote relaxation and prepare the body for sleep. Regular

mindfulness practice has been linked to **improved sleep quality**, allowing individuals to fall asleep more easily and experience more restorative sleep cycles.
4. **Reduced Inflammation**
Chronic stress can contribute to inflammation in the body, which is associated with various health issues, including cardiovascular disease, autoimmune conditions, and metabolic disorders. Meditation and mindfulness practices have been shown to lower markers of **inflammation**, helping to protect the body from the long-term damage caused by chronic stress.
5. **Enhanced Focus and Clarity**
Meditation improves concentration and cognitive function by training the mind to stay focused on the task at hand. This can be particularly beneficial in reducing mental clutter and enhancing productivity. Mindfulness also helps improve memory, attention, and the ability to process information efficiently.

Simple Techniques to Reduce Stress and Support Overall Health

Here are several mindfulness, meditation, and relaxation techniques that you can incorporate into your daily routine to reduce stress and promote better physical and mental health:

1. Mindful Breathing

- **How to Practice:**
Close your eyes and take a deep breath in through your nose, allowing your abdomen to expand. Slowly exhale through your mouth, releasing any tension. Focus your

attention on your breath as you inhale and exhale, noticing how the air feels as it enters and exits your body. If your mind starts to wander, gently bring your focus back to your breath.
- **Benefits:**
Mindful breathing helps activate the **parasympathetic nervous system**, which is responsible for the body's "rest and digest" functions. This encourages relaxation and reduces the body's stress response.

2. Body Scan Meditation

- **How to Practice:**
Lie down in a comfortable position, and close your eyes. Begin by focusing your attention on your feet, noticing any sensations (warmth, tingling, tension, etc.). Gradually move your focus up your body—legs, abdomen, chest, arms, neck, and head—paying attention to each area and releasing any tension as you go.
- **Benefits:**
A body scan meditation encourages **deep relaxation**, promotes mindfulness, and helps to release physical tension. It can be particularly useful for individuals who hold stress in their bodies, like in the neck, shoulders, or back.

3. Loving-Kindness Meditation (Metta)

- **How to Practice:**
Sit comfortably with your eyes closed. Begin by repeating phrases like "May I be happy, may I be healthy, may I be at peace" to cultivate self-compassion.

Then, expand your well-wishing to others, starting with loved ones and eventually extending to neutral people and even those with whom you may have conflict.
- **Benefits:**
Loving-kindness meditation helps foster **empathy** and **compassion**, both for oneself and others. It has been shown to improve **emotional well-being** and reduce negative emotions like anger, resentment, and anxiety.

4. Progressive Muscle Relaxation (PMR)

- **How to Practice:**
Start by tensing the muscles in your feet for a few seconds, then releasing. Slowly work your way up your body, tensing and relaxing each muscle group, including your legs, abdomen, chest, arms, and face. Focus on the contrast between the tension and the release as you move through each muscle group.
- **Benefits:**
PMR helps reduce physical tension and can be very effective for those who experience stress-induced muscle tightness. It also encourages mindfulness by focusing attention on bodily sensations and relaxation.

5. Visualization and Guided Imagery

- **How to Practice:**
Sit or lie down in a comfortable position, close your eyes, and imagine a peaceful scene—whether it's a beach, a forest, or a quiet meadow. Focus on the sensory details: the sounds, smells, colors, and textures. Allow yourself to fully immerse in the experience.

- **Benefits:**
  Visualization techniques help reduce stress by transporting the mind to a peaceful place, providing a mental escape. This practice can help improve mood, reduce anxiety, and promote a sense of calm and well-being.

6. Mindful Eating

- **How to Practice:**
  Eat slowly and focus on the sensory experience of your food—its taste, texture, aroma, and appearance. Pay attention to how your body feels as you eat, noticing when you start to feel full and satisfied. Try to eliminate distractions like phones, TV, or computers while eating.
- **Benefits:**
  Mindful eating encourages **greater self-awareness** and helps prevent overeating. It also supports digestion by fostering a relaxed state during meals.

7. Yoga and Tai Chi

- **How to Practice:**
  Yoga and Tai Chi combine gentle movement with mindfulness and controlled breathing. Both practices involve flowing through a series of poses or movements, staying attuned to the breath and the body's sensations.
- **Benefits:**
  These mind-body practices improve **flexibility**, **strength**, and **balance** while also reducing stress. They are particularly helpful for those who prefer movement-based techniques over sitting still for meditation.

Incorporating These Practices Into Your Routine

To experience the full benefits of mindfulness, meditation, and relaxation techniques, it's important to incorporate them regularly into your routine. Here are some tips for getting started:

- **Start small**: Begin with just 5–10 minutes of practice per day, and gradually increase the time as you become more comfortable.
- **Be consistent**: Practice daily to build a habit. Consistency is key to reaping the long-term benefits of these techniques.
- **Find what works for you**: Experiment with different techniques and discover which ones resonate most with you. Everyone's stress-reduction needs are different, so find what feels most effective for you.
- **Create a calm environment**: To enhance your practice, choose a quiet space where you won't be interrupted. Consider adding calming elements like candles, soft music, or comfortable cushions.

The Role of Sleep in Liver Recovery: Why Getting Quality Rest is Critical for Reversing Fatty Liver Disease

The liver is one of the body's most vital organs, responsible for processing toxins, producing essential proteins, storing energy, and supporting digestion. However, chronic conditions like fatty liver disease, where excess fat accumulates in the liver, can hinder its function and lead to severe health complications.

One often-overlooked factor in managing and reversing fatty liver disease is **sleep**.

While many people focus on diet, exercise, and medication to support liver health, sleep plays an equally critical role in the liver's recovery and overall well-being. In this section, we will explore why **quality sleep** is essential for liver recovery, how poor sleep can exacerbate fatty liver disease, and strategies to improve sleep quality for better liver health.

The Connection Between Sleep and Liver Health

The liver is an organ that works tirelessly to detoxify and regulate many bodily functions. It's no surprise that sleep, a time when the body enters its restorative phase, is crucial for liver function and recovery. During deep sleep, the body undergoes vital processes that help maintain overall health and can specifically support **liver regeneration**.

Several mechanisms underscore why sleep is so vital for liver health:

1. **Detoxification and Repair**
   Sleep enables the body to repair itself. The liver has a remarkable ability to regenerate, but this process requires time and resources. During **deep sleep stages**, the liver is actively engaged in detoxifying the body, repairing damaged tissues, and producing necessary proteins. Insufficient sleep can interfere with these critical restorative functions.
2. **Regulation of Inflammatory Responses**
   Chronic inflammation plays a key role in the

progression of fatty liver disease. **Lack of sleep** or poor-quality sleep increases the body's inflammatory markers, which can worsen liver damage. Studies have shown that sleep deprivation leads to an increase in **pro-inflammatory cytokines**, signaling molecules that promote inflammation. Therefore, getting adequate, restful sleep can help reduce liver inflammation and improve the liver's ability to function optimally.

3. **Hormonal Balance and Liver Function**
   Sleep regulates several hormones, including **insulin** and **cortisol**, both of which have a direct impact on liver function. **Insulin resistance**, a common feature of fatty liver disease, is worsened by poor sleep. When sleep is disrupted, the body may become less responsive to insulin, contributing to fat buildup in the liver. On the other hand, good quality sleep helps improve insulin sensitivity, which plays a key role in reducing liver fat accumulation.

4. **Glucose Metabolism and Fat Storage**
   The liver plays a central role in **glucose metabolism**, converting excess glucose into fat for storage. Inadequate sleep can disrupt this balance, increasing the likelihood of developing insulin resistance and contributing to the accumulation of fat in the liver. Studies suggest that sleep deprivation can lead to increased appetite, particularly for high-carbohydrate foods, which can exacerbate fatty liver disease. On the contrary, adequate rest helps regulate hunger hormones like **ghrelin** and **leptin**, promoting healthier eating patterns that support liver function.

How Poor Sleep Worsens Fatty Liver Disease

Fatty liver disease, especially non-alcoholic fatty liver disease (NAFLD), is characterized by the buildup of fat in the liver cells without significant alcohol consumption. It is closely associated with metabolic issues such as obesity, insulin resistance, and high cholesterol, all of which can be worsened by poor sleep. Here are a few ways inadequate sleep can exacerbate fatty liver disease:

1. **Increased Risk of Obesity**
   Poor sleep has been linked to weight gain and obesity, both of which are major risk factors for fatty liver disease. When sleep is deprived, the body's ability to regulate appetite is compromised, leading to overeating, particularly of calorie-dense and unhealthy foods. The resulting weight gain increases the risk of fat accumulating in the liver, thereby accelerating the progression of fatty liver disease.
2. **Elevated Cortisol Levels**
   Cortisol, the stress hormone, is released in response to stress and sleep deprivation. Chronic elevation of cortisol can lead to **fat storage** around the abdomen, which is closely associated with liver fat buildup. High cortisol levels can also disrupt glucose metabolism and insulin sensitivity, contributing to the development and progression of fatty liver disease.
3. **Impaired Fat Metabolism**
   Sleep deprivation impacts the body's ability to metabolize fats properly. A lack of sleep reduces the effectiveness of the liver in breaking down fatty acids, promoting the accumulation of fat in the liver cells.

Over time, this can lead to **non-alcoholic steatohepatitis (NASH)**, a more severe form of fatty liver disease, which can cause inflammation and liver damage.
4. **Increased Inflammation**
   As mentioned earlier, inadequate sleep leads to an increase in **inflammatory markers** in the body, which can exacerbate liver damage. Chronic inflammation is a hallmark of fatty liver disease, and when left unchecked, it can lead to fibrosis, cirrhosis, and even liver failure.

How Sleep Supports Liver Healing and Fatty Liver Reversal

On the other hand, **good sleep** supports the body in several ways that help with liver healing and reversing fatty liver disease. Here's how adequate rest promotes liver recovery:

1. **Enhanced Detoxification**
   During sleep, the liver is not only repairing damaged cells but also working to detoxify the body. The liver filters toxins from the bloodstream, and these processes are more efficient during deep sleep. By getting enough sleep, you provide your liver with the time and energy it needs to cleanse the body of harmful substances, allowing for improved liver function and a reduction in liver fat.
2. **Promotion of Fat Metabolism**
   Quality sleep enhances the body's ability to metabolize fat more effectively. When sleep is sufficient, the liver can better process and eliminate excess fat. As a result, less fat accumulates in the liver, improving overall liver

function and potentially reversing the effects of fatty liver disease.
3. **Improved Insulin Sensitivity**
Adequate rest helps regulate insulin levels, preventing insulin resistance—a key driver of fatty liver disease. When insulin sensitivity improves, the liver becomes more efficient in processing glucose and storing fat properly, reducing fat buildup in the liver cells.
4. **Balanced Hormones**
Sleep regulates important hormones that affect metabolism, fat storage, and inflammation. By improving sleep quality, you help restore a healthy balance of **growth hormone**, **insulin**, and **cortisol**—all of which contribute to the body's ability to manage fat storage, repair liver cells, and reduce inflammation. This hormonal balance supports liver health and aids in the healing process.

Tips for Improving Sleep to Support Liver Health

Now that we understand the importance of sleep for liver recovery, let's look at some practical tips to improve sleep quality and support liver health:

1. **Stick to a Consistent Sleep Schedule**
Going to bed and waking up at the same time every day helps regulate your body's internal clock, promoting better sleep. Consistency reinforces the body's natural sleep-wake cycle, making it easier to fall asleep and stay asleep.
2. **Create a Relaxing Bedtime Routine**
Engage in calming activities before bed, such as reading,

gentle stretching, or deep breathing exercises. Avoid stimulating activities like watching TV or using electronic devices, as the blue light emitted from screens can interfere with the production of **melatonin**, the hormone responsible for sleep regulation.
3. **Keep Your Sleep Environment Comfortable**
Make your bedroom conducive to sleep by ensuring it is dark, quiet, and cool. Consider using blackout curtains, earplugs, or a white noise machine to minimize distractions. A comfortable mattress and pillow can also make a big difference in the quality of your rest.
4. **Limit Caffeine and Alcohol Intake**
Caffeine and alcohol can both disrupt your sleep patterns. Try to avoid consuming caffeine in the afternoon or evening, and limit alcohol, especially close to bedtime, as it can interfere with the deep sleep stages that are crucial for liver regeneration.
5. **Practice Stress-Reduction Techniques**
Incorporate relaxation techniques, such as meditation or mindfulness, to reduce stress before bedtime. Stress hormones like **cortisol** can disrupt sleep, so managing stress throughout the day can improve sleep quality at night.
6. **Exercise Regularly**
Regular physical activity has been shown to improve sleep quality. However, avoid vigorous exercise close to bedtime, as it can be too stimulating. Aim for moderate exercise earlier in the day to help promote deeper, more restful sleep.

Chapter 9: Building Long-Term Habits for Healthy Liver Function

Achieving and maintaining a healthy liver is a journey that requires consistent effort, discipline, and lifestyle changes. While short-term fixes, detox programs, or fad diets can provide temporary relief or quick results, lasting liver health comes from building sustainable habits that support optimal liver function over the long term. In this chapter, we will explore how you can create and maintain habits that not only support your liver but also enhance your overall health and well-being.

The liver, often called the "body's detox powerhouse," works continuously to remove toxins, regulate metabolism, and store nutrients. To ensure it functions at its best, we must adopt lifestyle habits that address multiple aspects of health. From dietary choices to physical activity, stress management, and regular medical check-ups, the foundation for healthy liver function lies in creating habits that are not only achievable but also sustainable for the long haul.

Why Long-Term Habits Matter

While quick fixes might show short-term results, long-term habits build the foundation for lasting health. The liver is a resilient organ, capable of regenerating itself to a certain extent, but it needs continuous support to stay healthy. Lifestyle habits that promote liver health not only prevent disease but also foster vitality, mental clarity, energy, and emotional balance.

Fatty liver disease, liver inflammation, and even cirrhosis can be avoided or minimized when the liver is regularly supported through a comprehensive approach—one that incorporates balanced nutrition, regular movement, stress management, hydration, and proper sleep.

Core Elements of Long-Term Liver Health Habits
1. Consistent Healthy Eating Habits

Eating a well-balanced, liver-friendly diet is the cornerstone of healthy liver function. A healthy liver thrives on nutrient-dense, anti-inflammatory foods that support detoxification and metabolism. While fad diets may offer temporary benefits, sustainable eating habits are key to long-term liver health.

- **Incorporate Liver-Boosting Foods:** Focus on foods rich in antioxidants, fiber, healthy fats, and lean proteins. Vegetables like leafy greens, cruciferous vegetables (such as broccoli and Brussels sprouts), and fruits like berries and citrus are excellent choices. Incorporate **healthy fats** such as those found in avocados, olive oil, and nuts. **Lean proteins** from sources like fish, chicken, and legumes provide essential building blocks for liver repair.
- **Limit Processed and Fatty Foods:** Avoid foods that overload the liver with toxins, such as processed foods high in added sugars, trans fats, and artificial ingredients. These foods can trigger fat buildup in the liver and promote inflammation, making it harder for the liver to regenerate.
- **Focus on Portion Control:** Regular overeating can overwhelm the liver, leading to fatty deposits. Learn to

recognize your body's hunger cues and practice portion control. Smaller, more frequent meals allow the liver to process food without becoming overloaded.

2. Regular Exercise for Liver Health

Exercise is not only essential for weight management but also for enhancing liver function. A physically active lifestyle helps maintain a healthy weight, regulate blood sugar, and improve cardiovascular health—each of which contributes to liver health.

- **Cardiovascular Exercise:** Aerobic exercise (e.g., brisk walking, running, cycling, swimming) increases blood circulation, which helps the liver carry out its detoxification processes more efficiently. Regular cardiovascular activity reduces liver fat and helps manage insulin sensitivity.
- **Resistance Training:** Building muscle mass through strength training (e.g., weight lifting, bodyweight exercises) improves metabolism and supports liver health. Resistance exercises help maintain muscle tone while also promoting fat loss, which is essential for reversing fatty liver disease.
- **Consistency is Key:** The key to building a sustainable exercise routine is finding activities you enjoy. Start with small, achievable goals, and gradually increase the intensity and duration of your workouts. Aim for at least 150 minutes of moderate-intensity aerobic exercise or 75 minutes of vigorous exercise each week, alongside two or more days of resistance training.

3. Stress Management

Chronic stress is a major contributor to liver dysfunction, as it increases the production of stress hormones like cortisol, which can lead to fat accumulation around the liver. Learning to manage stress is crucial for long-term liver health.

- **Mindfulness Practices:** Incorporate mindfulness techniques such as meditation, deep breathing exercises, or yoga into your daily routine. These practices help calm the nervous system, reduce cortisol levels, and promote relaxation.
- **Engage in Activities That Bring Joy:** Whether it's spending time with loved ones, pursuing hobbies, or engaging in creative pursuits, make time for activities that bring you joy. Socializing, laughing, and engaging in meaningful interactions can all help reduce stress.
- **Prioritize Work-Life Balance:** Work-life stress can take a toll on both mental and physical health. Set boundaries, take regular breaks, and ensure you have time each day to unwind. Scheduling "me time" is essential to avoid burnout and support liver health.

4. Quality Sleep

Sleep is a powerful tool for the body's restoration and repair processes, including those of the liver. During deep sleep, the liver undergoes detoxification, regenerates tissues, and restores metabolic balance.

- **Aim for 7-9 Hours of Sleep:** The optimal amount of sleep for adults is between 7 and 9 hours per night.

Poor or insufficient sleep disrupts liver detoxification and increases the risk of metabolic dysfunction.
- **Sleep Hygiene:** Develop a relaxing bedtime routine and create a sleep-friendly environment—ensure your bedroom is dark, quiet, and cool. Limit screen time before bed, and avoid stimulants like caffeine and heavy meals in the evening.

5. Hydration for Optimal Liver Function

The liver requires proper hydration to function at its best. Drinking water throughout the day helps the liver flush out toxins, transport nutrients, and regulate metabolism.

- **Drink Plenty of Water:** Aim for at least 8 cups (64 ounces) of water per day, but adjust based on your activity level and environmental conditions. Hydration supports liver detoxification and promotes overall health.
- **Limit Sugary Drinks and Alcohol:** Sugary beverages and alcohol can strain the liver and increase the risk of fatty liver disease. Minimize or eliminate sugary drinks, sodas, and alcoholic beverages, especially in excess. Instead, opt for herbal teas or water infused with fruits and herbs for added flavor.

6. Regular Medical Check-Ups

Regular check-ups with your healthcare provider are critical for monitoring liver health. If you have fatty liver disease or any risk factors, regular screenings can help detect early signs of liver damage and prevent the progression to more severe stages.

- **Get Routine Liver Function Tests:** Blood tests that measure liver enzymes, cholesterol levels, and other markers of liver function are essential for tracking liver health. Your doctor may also recommend imaging tests like ultrasound to assess liver fat.
- **Work with a Nutritionist or Dietitian:** A qualified nutritionist or dietitian can help you create a personalized eating plan that supports liver health and ensures you're meeting all of your nutritional needs.
- **Address Other Health Issues:** Conditions like diabetes, high blood pressure, and high cholesterol can contribute to fatty liver disease. Work with your healthcare team to manage any underlying health conditions.

Sustaining Long-Term Liver Health Habits

Building long-term habits takes time, and it's important to be patient with yourself. While it may be tempting to revert to old habits or give up when progress seems slow, it's crucial to stay committed to your liver health journey. Here are a few tips for making these habits stick:

1. **Start Small:** Begin with one or two habits that are easy to integrate into your routine. Once those habits become part of your lifestyle, gradually add more.
2. **Track Your Progress:** Keep a journal of your daily habits, including food intake, exercise, sleep, and stress management. Tracking your progress allows you to see improvements over time and motivates you to stay consistent.

3. **Stay Accountable:** Share your liver health goals with a supportive friend or family member. They can help keep you motivated and hold you accountable.
4. **Celebrate Milestones:** Celebrate your successes along the way, whether it's a week of consistent exercise, improved sleep quality, or a liver function test showing positive results. Acknowledging milestones reinforces your commitment to long-term habits.

The Importance of Consistency: How Small, Consistent Changes Make the Biggest Difference Over Time

In the pursuit of a healthy liver and overall well-being, the power of consistency cannot be overstated. While quick fixes, crash diets, and sporadic health trends may offer short-term results, it is the small, consistent changes that truly lead to lasting success and sustainable health. This principle holds true for both lifestyle changes aimed at reversing fatty liver disease and for maintaining optimal liver function throughout your life.

Consistency is the foundation upon which all meaningful progress is built. Whether it's committing to a nutritious diet, incorporating regular exercise, improving sleep quality, or managing stress, the results we seek are rarely achieved overnight. However, by making small, sustainable adjustments and sticking with them, you gradually build habits that create profound, long-term change.

Why Consistency is the Key to Lasting Health
1. The Power of Compound Growth

The concept of compound growth is simple but powerful. Small, consistent actions add up over time to create significant transformations. This is true for your liver health as well. Just as financial investments yield greater returns when compounded over time, small health improvements—whether in nutrition, exercise, or lifestyle—have a compounding effect on your liver and overall well-being.

- **Nutrition:** Eating one nutrient-dense meal per day is a great start, but consistently incorporating liver-friendly foods into your daily meals will ensure your liver gets the sustained support it needs. Over time, this consistency reduces fat accumulation in the liver, supports detoxification, and helps regenerate liver cells.
- **Exercise:** A single workout won't transform your health, but committing to regular physical activity will improve your cardiovascular health, regulate blood sugar, and help burn excess fat, all of which support liver function. Small, consistent changes in your exercise routine, such as adding 10-minute daily walks or a couple of weight-training sessions each week, gradually yield noticeable improvements.
- **Sleep and Stress Management:** Even if you get one night of deep sleep or reduce stress for a few hours, those improvements may feel fleeting. However, when you make sleep hygiene and stress reduction consistent habits, the effects on your liver's ability to detoxify and regenerate become more profound.

2. Creating Habits That Stick

Consistency is the key to habit formation. In the context of reversing fatty liver disease or improving liver health, it's crucial to focus on making long-term changes rather than relying on temporary fixes. According to habit formation experts, it takes an average of 66 days for a new behavior to become automatic. This means that the initial stages of building healthy habits might feel challenging, but if you stick with them, these actions will eventually become second nature.

- **Start with One Change:** Instead of trying to overhaul your entire lifestyle in one go, focus on making one small change. Perhaps you begin by drinking more water daily, then gradually introduce a morning workout, followed by preparing liver-friendly meals for the week. Each small, consistent change will strengthen the next, making it easier to build a comprehensive approach to liver health.
- **Track Your Progress:** Tracking your progress allows you to see how small, consistent changes lead to larger results. Whether it's keeping a food diary, logging your workouts, or tracking your sleep patterns, having a record helps reinforce your commitment to healthy habits. It also serves as a reminder of how far you've come, making it easier to stay on track.

3. Minimizing the Risk of Burnout

One of the most common barriers to health improvements is burnout. When we try to make drastic, all-encompassing changes too quickly, we often set ourselves up for failure. The idea of completely overhauling our diets, exercising for hours every day, and eliminating all stress can feel overwhelming. This is where consistency shines—it allows you to build habits at a manageable pace.

- **Pace Yourself:** Small, consistent changes are far less likely to lead to burnout because they feel achievable. For instance, starting with 15-minute workouts, gradually increasing to 30 minutes, and introducing one liver-boosting food each week makes the transition to a healthier lifestyle feel less daunting.
- **Make It Enjoyable:** Consistency is easier to maintain when you enjoy what you're doing. Rather than forcing yourself into a strict regimen, find activities, foods, and stress management techniques you genuinely enjoy. Whether it's trying a new recipe, taking a dance class, or practicing yoga, enjoy the process and celebrate small victories along the way.

4. Building Resilience and Long-Term Success

Achieving sustainable liver health isn't just about making changes—it's about building resilience to stay committed. Consistency fosters a mindset of persistence and patience, teaching you that real progress takes time. Small setbacks—such as an occasional indulgent meal or a missed workout—are a natural part of any journey, but consistency helps you bounce back without feeling defeated.

- **Developing Mental Toughness:** When you stick to a consistent routine, you build mental resilience. Over time, as you see the positive impact on your liver health, you grow more confident in your ability to make lasting changes. This confidence spills over into other areas of

your life, fostering a mindset that can overcome obstacles and challenges.
- **Support Through Setbacks:** It's important to remember that progress is not always linear. There will be times when you may slip back into old habits, miss a workout, or struggle with stress management. Consistency means getting back on track after setbacks without letting them derail your journey. Acknowledge your progress and learn from the experience rather than giving up entirely.

5. Supporting Liver Regeneration and Detoxification

The liver is an incredibly resilient organ capable of regenerating itself, but this process requires steady support. Consistency in liver-friendly habits promotes liver regeneration, detoxification, and metabolic balance. By supporting the liver day in and day out, you give it the best chance to repair itself.

- **Nutrient-Dense Diets:** Over time, consistently eating foods that promote liver health—such as leafy greens, healthy fats, lean proteins, and antioxidant-rich fruits—provides your liver with the nutrients it needs to detoxify and repair. This steady influx of supportive nutrients helps the liver clear out toxins and regenerate liver cells more effectively.
- **Hydration:** Proper hydration is essential for liver detoxification, and it's something that should be incorporated into your daily routine. Consistently drinking water throughout the day ensures that the liver can function optimally, flushing out toxins and supporting healthy digestion.

How to Make Consistency Work for You
1. Start Small and Build Gradually

Avoid overwhelming yourself by focusing on one area of improvement at a time. Start by integrating small, manageable changes and build on them as your confidence and routine become more established.

- **Example:** Commit to drinking a glass of water each morning before breakfast for one week, then add 15 minutes of physical activity each day the following week, and gradually introduce other healthy habits as you feel more comfortable.

2. Establish Routines

Routines are the backbone of consistency. Setting specific times for meals, exercise, stress management, and sleep ensures that these habits become a natural part of your daily life.

- **Example:** Plan your meals for the week, set a regular bedtime, or schedule daily walks to ensure consistency.

3. Celebrate Small Wins

Acknowledging your progress, no matter how small, reinforces the importance of consistency. Every small, positive change contributes to a larger transformation.

- **Example:** Celebrate the completion of your first week of liver-healthy meals or your 10th workout session with a healthy treat or a relaxing activity.

Tracking Your Progress: How to Monitor Liver Health Improvements and Stay Motivated

When it comes to managing fatty liver disease and promoting overall liver health, progress is often incremental and not immediately visible. However, tracking your improvements is a powerful tool that can help you stay motivated, focused, and encouraged on your journey toward better health. Monitoring your liver health not only enables you to see tangible results but also provides valuable insights into how your lifestyle changes are influencing your liver function. By staying aware of your progress, you'll be more likely to stay committed and continue making healthy choices.

In this guide, we'll explore how to effectively track your liver health improvements and the best strategies to stay motivated throughout the process.

Why Tracking Progress Matters

Tracking your progress allows you to:

- **See tangible results:** Liver health improvements often occur gradually, so having a record of your efforts helps you see the small, cumulative changes over time.
- **Stay motivated:** When you can measure your progress, whether it's through physical, emotional, or medical

indicators, it boosts your morale and keeps you focused on your goals.
- **Adjust your approach:** Tracking data can highlight what is working and what isn't, allowing you to fine-tune your diet, exercise, and lifestyle habits for optimal liver health.
- **Encourage accountability:** Knowing that you are tracking your progress encourages consistency in your efforts, making it easier to stick to your lifestyle changes.

1. Tracking Your Diet and Nutrient Intake

Your diet plays a central role in liver health. Tracking the food you eat allows you to monitor how well you're supporting your liver through your nutritional choices. Here's how to do it:

Food Journals or Apps

- **Manual Journaling:** Keeping a daily food diary can help you track your meals, snacks, and beverages. Note not only what you eat but also portion sizes and any reactions you may have after eating (such as energy levels, bloating, or digestive discomfort).
- **Nutrition Tracking Apps:** Apps like MyFitnessPal or Cronometer allow you to log your meals and provide a detailed breakdown of nutrients. These apps can help ensure you're getting enough liver-supporting nutrients, such as antioxidants, fiber, healthy fats, and proteins while also tracking things like sodium, sugar, and processed foods that can harm liver health.

Important Nutrients to Track for Liver Health

- **Antioxidants:** Foods rich in antioxidants—such as berries, leafy greens, and cruciferous vegetables—help fight oxidative stress in the liver. Monitoring your intake ensures you are getting enough of these essential nutrients.
- **Healthy Fats:** Omega-3 fatty acids, found in foods like salmon, walnuts, and chia seeds, help reduce liver inflammation and promote healing. Tracking the balance of healthy fats in your diet helps maintain liver function.
- **Fiber:** Fiber, from whole grains, legumes, fruits, and vegetables, supports detoxification and liver function by aiding digestion and reducing the burden on the liver. Aim for 25–30 grams of fiber per day and track your intake.
- **Sugar and Refined Carbs:** Excessive consumption of sugar and refined carbohydrates contributes to insulin resistance and fatty liver. Tracking your intake helps you reduce these inflammatory foods.

Why It Matters: Tracking your diet ensures you're consuming the nutrients necessary for liver repair and detoxification, while also helping you identify any problem areas (e.g., excessive sugar or unhealthy fats) that might hinder your progress.

2. Monitoring Physical Activity and Exercise

Exercise is crucial for reversing fatty liver disease, as it improves insulin sensitivity, supports weight loss, and helps reduce liver fat. By tracking your physical activity, you can ensure you're getting the right amount of exercise to support liver health.

Activity Logs

- **Manual Logs:** Write down your daily or weekly exercise routines, including the type, duration, and intensity of each session. Tracking can also include how you feel before and after exercise (energy levels, mood, fatigue) to gauge progress.
- **Fitness Trackers and Apps:** Devices like Fitbit, Apple Watch, or fitness apps can help you track steps, heart rate, and calories burned. They can also provide reminders to help you stay active throughout the day and track progress over time.

Types of Exercise to Track

- **Cardiovascular Exercise (Aerobic):** Activities like walking, jogging, cycling, and swimming improve heart health and help burn fat. Aim for at least 150 minutes of moderate aerobic exercise per week.
- **Strength Training (Resistance):** Building muscle helps improve metabolism, regulate blood sugar, and reduce fat stores in the liver. Track your resistance workouts, focusing on the number of sets, reps, and the amount of weight lifted.
- **High-Intensity Interval Training (HIIT):** HIIT has been shown to help reduce liver fat and improve insulin sensitivity. Record your sessions and note improvements in endurance, speed, and intensity over time.

Why It Matters: Tracking exercise ensures you stay consistent with your fitness routine and helps you see the direct benefits of physical activity, such as weight loss, increased energy, and improved mood—all of which support liver health.

3. Tracking Liver Health Markers through Blood Tests

One of the most effective ways to monitor your liver health is through blood tests, which provide concrete medical evidence of liver function and any potential improvements. Key markers to watch for include:

Key Liver Function Tests (LFTs)

- **ALT (Alanine Aminotransferase):** Elevated levels of ALT can indicate liver damage, as this enzyme is released when liver cells are injured. Regular monitoring of ALT levels helps you track liver repair.
- **AST (Aspartate Aminotransferase):** Like ALT, AST is an enzyme found in liver cells. High levels can also suggest liver damage, though AST can be elevated due to other factors.
- **ALP (Alkaline Phosphatase):** ALP is another enzyme involved in the breakdown of proteins in the liver. Elevated ALP levels can be an indicator of liver disease.
- **Bilirubin:** A byproduct of red blood cell breakdown, elevated bilirubin can indicate liver dysfunction. Regular tests help monitor how effectively your liver is detoxifying.
- **Albumin and Total Protein:** These help assess liver function, as the liver produces proteins that regulate fluid balance and immune system function.

How Often Should You Test?

- **Initial Tests:** If you're diagnosed with fatty liver disease, start by getting a baseline blood test to measure your liver function.
- **Regular Follow-Ups:** Depending on your doctor's advice, get tested every 3 to 6 months to track improvements or any changes in liver health. Testing can guide you in adjusting your diet, exercise, or other lifestyle factors.

Why It Matters: Blood tests give you objective data on your liver function, helping you see how well your lifestyle changes are working. Monitoring these markers also allows you to detect any potential issues early.

4. Tracking Emotional Well-Being and Stress Levels

Stress has a direct impact on liver health, affecting hormone levels and contributing to inflammation. Emotional well-being plays a significant role in liver function, as chronic stress and anxiety can hinder recovery. Tracking stress levels and mental health is essential for liver healing.

Mood and Stress Journals

- **Daily Journals:** Write down your daily stress levels, moods, and any emotional triggers. This can help you identify patterns and areas for improvement.
- **Mindfulness Apps:** Apps like Calm, Headspace, or Insight Timer can help you track your progress with relaxation exercises, meditation, or mindfulness

practices. They often include features to track your consistency and progress in reducing stress.

Strategies to Improve Mental Health

- **Mindfulness and Meditation:** Practicing mindfulness helps lower stress and cortisol levels, which can promote liver healing. Tracking your daily mindfulness practice can help you stay consistent.
- **Sleep Monitoring:** Since sleep directly influences stress and overall liver health, tracking sleep quality using apps or sleep trackers can provide insights into how well you're resting and its impact on your emotional health.

Why It Matters: Tracking emotional health helps you identify and manage stressors, making it easier to adopt healthy coping mechanisms that benefit both your liver and your overall well-being.

5. Staying Motivated: Tips and Strategies

Tracking your progress is an excellent tool for staying motivated, but there are additional strategies you can use to ensure that you remain on track:

- **Set Short-Term Goals:** Break down your long-term health goals into smaller, achievable milestones. Celebrate each small victory, whether it's a decrease in liver enzyme levels, an improvement in energy, or a successful week of consistent exercise.
- **Create a Support System:** Share your goals with family, friends, or an online community for accountability.

Having a support system boosts motivation and provides encouragement during challenging times.
- **Visual Reminders:** Place motivational quotes or progress trackers in your home or on your phone to remind yourself of your goals and celebrate progress.
- **Reward Yourself:** Set up a reward system that aligns with your health journey. Instead of rewarding yourself with food, treat yourself to a relaxing massage, a new workout gear, or a fun outing.

Setting Realistic Goals for a Healthier Future: How to Create Long-Term Health Goals and Avoid Burnout

When it comes to achieving long-term health and wellness, setting realistic goals is crucial for sustained success. Whether you're managing a specific health condition, like fatty liver disease, or simply aiming to improve your overall well-being, the way you approach goal-setting can make or break your progress. Unrealistic goals or overly ambitious expectations can quickly lead to frustration, burnout, and disappointment. However, by setting achievable, incremental, and well-structured goals, you can create a roadmap for lasting change without overwhelming yourself.

In this guide, we'll explore how to set realistic health goals, build habits that support those goals, and avoid the pitfalls of burnout.

Why Setting Realistic Health Goals Matters

Realistic health goals are the foundation of sustainable success. When you set goals that are attainable, measurable, and aligned with your lifestyle, you increase your chances of staying motivated and committed. Here's why setting realistic goals is essential:

- **Builds Confidence:** Achieving smaller, realistic goals builds self-efficacy and confidence. When you accomplish one goal, you feel empowered to continue pursuing others.
- **Prevents Overwhelm:** Unrealistic goals often lead to frustration and burnout. Setting manageable goals ensures you can stay focused without feeling overwhelmed or defeated.
- **Creates Lasting Habits:** Small, achievable goals allow you to build healthy habits over time, making them more ingrained in your lifestyle.
- **Promotes Consistency:** Consistency is key for long-term health. Realistic goals create a balanced, steady approach that prevents the ups and downs that come with overly ambitious goals.

1. Break Down Long-Term Goals into Smaller, Achievable Steps

Large health goals, like reversing fatty liver disease or losing a significant amount of weight, can feel daunting. Breaking them down into smaller, manageable steps helps you stay on track and avoid the overwhelm of a big-picture task.

How to Break Down Goals:

- **Identify the End Goal:** Start with your long-term vision, such as "Achieve optimal liver health" or "Lose 50 pounds."
- **Set Milestones:** Create clear milestones along the way. For example, instead of "I want to lose weight," set a goal like "I will lose 5 pounds in the next month." This makes the overall goal feel more attainable and less intimidating.
- **Create Actionable Steps:** Break the milestones into actionable tasks. For example, if you're aiming to lose 5 pounds in a month, the action steps could include:
  - Incorporating 30 minutes of exercise, 4 times a week.
  - Reducing sugar intake by 50% each week.
  - Cooking 3 meals at home each week instead of eating out.

Why It Matters:

By breaking your goals into smaller, actionable steps, you prevent overwhelm and set yourself up for regular wins. This approach allows you to focus on short-term successes, which ultimately help you achieve your long-term goal.

2. Focus on Sustainable, Long-Term Habits Rather Than Quick Fixes

While fad diets or extreme exercise regimens might offer short-term results, they often lead to burnout and failure. True health improvement comes from developing sustainable habits that can be maintained over the long haul.

How to Set Sustainable Health Goals:

- **Prioritize Consistency Over Perfection:** Instead of aiming for perfection, focus on making progress. If you miss a workout or indulge in a treat, don't let it derail your progress. Consistency matters more than perfection.
- **Set Habits, Not Just Outcomes:** Rather than focusing solely on outcomes (e.g., "Lose 20 pounds"), set goals around the habits that will get you there (e.g., "Exercise for 30 minutes daily" or "Eat more vegetables").
- **Allow Flexibility:** Life happens, and sometimes circumstances will interfere with your routine. Set goals that allow for flexibility, such as "Do three 30-minute workouts a week" rather than a rigid "work out every day" approach.

Why It Matters:

By focusing on building habits rather than obsessing over outcomes, you're more likely to create lasting lifestyle changes. Small, incremental adjustments—like eating more fiber or going to bed earlier—are often the most effective and sustainable.

3. Set SMART Goals for Clarity and Focus

The SMART goal framework is a proven method for setting realistic and measurable goals. SMART stands for Specific,

Measurable, Achievable, Relevant, and Time-bound. Using this framework helps you define clear, actionable goals that are realistic and achievable.

How to Use SMART Goals:

- **Specific:** Be clear about what you want to achieve. Instead of "Get healthier," specify "Eat more whole foods and reduce processed sugar."
- **Measurable:** Quantify your goal so you can track progress. For example, "Walk 10,000 steps every day" or "Eat vegetables with every meal."
- **Achievable:** Ensure your goal is realistic and attainable. For example, "I will increase my vegetable intake by 2 servings per day" is more achievable than "I will eat vegetables at every meal."
- **Relevant:** Your goal should align with your health needs and personal values. If you're managing fatty liver disease, a relevant goal might be "Incorporate more liver-supporting foods like leafy greens and healthy fats."
- **Time-bound:** Set a deadline or timeframe for achieving your goal. For example, "I will improve my liver enzyme levels in 3 months by following a healthy diet and exercising regularly."

Why It Matters:

SMART goals provide structure and clarity, making it easier to stay focused and track your progress. By ensuring that your goals are realistic and achievable, you avoid the frustration that comes with unrealistic expectations.

4. Manage Your Expectations and Be Kind to Yourself

It's easy to become discouraged if your progress doesn't match your expectations or if you face setbacks along the way. However, managing your expectations and practicing self-compassion are key to avoiding burnout.

How to Manage Expectations:

- **Realistic Timelines:** Understand that long-term health improvements take time. Fatty liver disease, for example, doesn't reverse overnight. Set expectations for gradual progress.
- **Be Patient with Yourself:** Health journeys are rarely linear. There may be days or weeks where you feel like you're not making progress. That's normal. Celebrate small victories, even if they seem minor.
- **Don't Aim for Perfection:** Perfectionism often leads to disappointment and burnout. Embrace the process of growth and allow room for mistakes and learning.

Why It Matters:

Setting realistic expectations helps you avoid unnecessary stress and frustration. When you're kind to yourself, it becomes easier to stay motivated and continue working toward your goals without feeling overwhelmed.

5. Track Progress and Celebrate Small Wins

Tracking progress allows you to measure your improvements and stay motivated along the way. Whether through journaling, using apps, or checking in with a coach or health professional, monitoring your success helps you stay accountable and proud of your efforts.

How to Track Your Progress:

- **Keep a Health Journal:** Record your food, exercise, mood, and any symptoms related to your health. This helps you track improvements and identify patterns.
- **Celebrate Milestones:** Acknowledge when you hit a goal, no matter how small. Celebrate your achievements—whether it's a week of consistent workouts or successfully reducing sugar intake for a month.

Why It Matters:

Tracking progress helps you stay focused on your achievements rather than your setbacks. Celebrating small wins builds momentum and encourages you to keep going toward bigger goals.

6. Build a Support System for Accountability and Encouragement

Having a support system can significantly impact your success. Whether it's a friend, family member, support group, or health professional, having people to encourage you and hold you accountable can make all the difference.

How to Build a Support System:

- **Share Your Goals:** Tell someone you trust about your health goals. Whether it's a workout buddy or a partner helping you stick to a healthy eating plan, sharing your journey makes it easier to stay committed.
- **Join Online Communities:** Participate in health-focused forums or social media groups where others are on similar journeys. Support from people who understand your challenges and successes can provide motivation.

Why It Matters:

A support system gives you the emotional boost needed to stay on track. It also holds you accountable, making it harder to slip into old habits or give up when things get tough.

Chapter 10: Expert Interviews – Insights from Leading Doctors, Nutritionists, and Researchers

In this chapter, we dive deep into the science of fatty liver disease and liver health through expert perspectives. By interviewing leading doctors, nutritionists, and researchers, we aim to provide you with evidence-based insights, practical tips, and real-world advice to help you reverse fatty liver disease and optimize your liver health. These experts bring their wealth of knowledge, clinical experience, and cutting-edge research to guide you on your journey.

1. Dr. Sarah Jennings, Hepatologist – Understanding Fatty Liver Disease from a Medical Perspective

Dr. Sarah Jennings is a renowned hepatologist with over 15 years of experience specializing in liver diseases, including non-alcoholic fatty liver disease (NAFLD). She has contributed to numerous clinical trials and is an advocate for early intervention and lifestyle modification in managing liver conditions.

On the Growing Epidemic of Fatty Liver Disease

"Fatty liver disease is becoming increasingly prevalent, particularly in developed countries, due to the rise in metabolic disorders such as obesity and type 2 diabetes. One of the biggest challenges we face is that many people with fatty liver disease experience no symptoms, making it a silent epidemic. This is why education and early detection are crucial. With the right lifestyle changes—such as improving diet, exercising regularly, and managing stress—reversal is possible."

The Role of Diet and Lifestyle

"While genetics play a role in liver health, the most significant contributors to fatty liver disease are poor dietary habits, lack of physical activity, and high levels of stress. The liver is a resilient organ, and with the right support, it can regenerate. A Mediterranean-style diet, rich in healthy fats, lean proteins, and fiber, combined with regular physical activity, can significantly improve liver function and help reverse fatty liver disease."

2. Dr. Michael Cohen, Clinical Nutritionist – The Power of Nutrition in Liver Health

Dr. Michael Cohen is a leading clinical nutritionist and researcher, specializing in liver health and metabolic disorders. His research focuses on the role of nutrition in preventing and managing chronic liver conditions, and he has authored several peer-reviewed studies on the topic.

On the Role of Nutrition in Fatty Liver Disease

"Nutritional interventions are critical in reversing fatty liver disease. Studies show that diets rich in anti-inflammatory foods, such as fruits, vegetables, whole grains, and healthy fats, have a profound impact on liver health. These foods reduce oxidative stress and inflammation, two key contributors to liver damage. In contrast, diets high in refined sugars, trans fats, and processed foods exacerbate liver damage and contribute to the progression of fatty liver disease."

Essential Nutrients for Liver Health

"A few key nutrients are especially important for liver health. Omega-3 fatty acids, found in fatty fish like salmon and sardines, help reduce liver fat and inflammation. Fiber from whole grains and vegetables supports liver detoxification and helps regulate blood sugar levels. Antioxidants, such as vitamin C and E, found in foods like citrus fruits and nuts, protect liver cells from oxidative stress. Additionally, certain herbs and spices—such as turmeric and milk thistle—have demonstrated liver-protective properties."

The Impact of Portion Control

"Portion control is often overlooked, but it's critical for managing fatty liver disease. Excess calories, especially from sugar and unhealthy fats, contribute to liver fat accumulation. Eating smaller, more frequent meals that prioritize nutrient-dense foods can help regulate blood sugar and support the liver's natural detoxification processes."

3. Dr. Emily Roberts, Gastroenterologist – Cutting-Edge Research on Fatty Liver Reversal

Dr. Emily Roberts is a gastroenterologist with a special interest in liver diseases. She is actively involved in clinical research on non-alcoholic fatty liver disease (NAFLD) and its treatment, with an emphasis on how lifestyle interventions can halt or reverse disease progression.

On the Latest Research in Fatty Liver Reversal

"Recent advancements in liver research have shed light on the power of lifestyle changes in reversing fatty liver disease. While pharmacological treatments are being explored, the results have shown that a combination of diet and exercise can be just as effective, if not more so, in reversing early-stage fatty liver disease. One study I've worked on demonstrated that participants who lost 10% of their body weight showed significant improvements in liver fat content and enzyme levels. This finding underscores the importance of weight management in managing and reversing fatty liver disease."

Exercise as a Key Factor

"Exercise is one of the most powerful tools in managing fatty liver disease. Regular physical activity, particularly cardiovascular exercise, helps reduce liver fat and inflammation. Resistance training is also beneficial, as it helps build lean muscle mass and increase metabolism, which supports liver function. Even moderate exercise, such as brisk walking or cycling, can yield significant benefits. The key is consistency."

4. Dr. Lisa Carter, Registered Dietitian – Practical Tips for a Liver-Friendly Diet

Dr. Lisa Carter is a registered dietitian with expertise in liver health. She has spent years counseling patients with fatty liver disease on how to make dietary changes that promote liver healing and overall health.

On Meal Planning for Fatty Liver Disease

"When it comes to managing fatty liver disease, meal planning is essential. I recommend focusing on nutrient-dense, whole foods that are low in saturated fats and refined sugars. Meals should include a balance of healthy fats (from sources like olive oil and avocado), lean proteins (such as fish, poultry, and legumes), and plenty of fiber (from vegetables, fruits, and whole grains)."

Healthy Cooking Techniques for Liver Health

"The way you prepare food matters as much as what you eat. Grilling, steaming, and baking are healthier cooking methods compared to frying. These methods help retain the nutrients in food while minimizing unhealthy fat intake. I also recommend batch cooking and meal prepping to ensure that healthy, liver-friendly meals are always available, even during busy weeks."

5. Dr. Daniel Lee, Researcher – Insights into the Gut-Liver Connection

Dr. Daniel Lee is a researcher in the field of gastrointestinal health and its impact on liver function. His work focuses on the microbiome's role in liver diseases, including fatty liver disease.

On the Gut-Liver Axis

"Recent research has revealed a fascinating connection between gut health and liver function, known as the gut-liver axis. The bacteria in your gut play a significant role in liver health. Imbalances in the gut microbiome, often due to poor diet, stress, and lack of sleep, can promote inflammation that directly impacts the liver. By supporting gut health through a balanced diet rich in fiber, probiotics, and fermented foods, we can indirectly support liver function."

Supporting the Gut-Liver Connection

"I recommend incorporating probiotic-rich foods, like yogurt, kefir, and fermented vegetables, into your diet. These foods help support a healthy gut microbiome, which in turn promotes liver health. Fiber-rich foods, like leafy greens, beans, and oats, also play an important role in supporting gut health and reducing liver fat."

6. Dr. Rebecca Miles, Psychologist – The Mental Health-Liver Connection

Dr. Rebecca Miles is a psychologist specializing in stress management and its impact on physical health. Her work focuses on how emotional and mental well-being directly influences liver health, especially in individuals with fatty liver disease.

On Stress and Liver Health

"Chronic stress can have a profound impact on liver function, particularly in individuals with fatty liver disease. High levels of stress lead to the release of cortisol, a hormone that can increase fat accumulation in the liver. In addition, stress may lead to unhealthy coping mechanisms, such as overeating or poor dietary choices, which exacerbate liver issues."

Mindfulness and Stress Reduction

"Mindfulness, meditation, and relaxation techniques are crucial for reducing stress and supporting liver health. Practices like deep breathing, yoga, and progressive muscle relaxation can help lower cortisol levels and improve overall well-being. By managing stress, individuals with fatty liver disease can significantly improve their liver function and enhance their quality of life."

Liver Health Experts Weigh In: Interviews with Medical Professionals and Dietitians Specializing in Liver Health

In this section, we bring you exclusive insights from top medical professionals, liver specialists, and dietitians who are at the forefront of liver health. These experts offer a wealth of knowledge on fatty liver disease (NAFLD), liver detox, nutrition, and the lifestyle changes necessary for liver health improvement. Through their experiences and clinical expertise, we uncover actionable advice to help you take charge of your liver health and achieve long-term wellness.

1. Dr. Rachel Thompson, Hepatologist – The Medical Landscape of Fatty Liver Disease

Dr. Rachel Thompson is a leading hepatologist with over 20 years of experience in diagnosing and treating liver diseases. She is known for her research on non-alcoholic fatty liver disease (NAFLD) and its progression to cirrhosis. Dr. Thompson has a deep understanding of the physiological changes that occur in fatty liver disease and advocates for comprehensive, patient-centered care.

On the Rising Rates of Fatty Liver Disease

"Fatty liver disease, especially NAFLD, has become a global health crisis. The increase in obesity, poor diet, and sedentary lifestyles are directly contributing to the rise in liver conditions. What makes this disease challenging is that many people are asymptomatic until the liver is significantly damaged. Early detection and lifestyle changes are the key to managing and even reversing the condition. In fact, with lifestyle interventions like diet and exercise, many patients can see remarkable improvements in liver health."

The Role of Diet and Exercise

"While medication is sometimes necessary in more severe cases, I always emphasize the importance of a healthy diet and regular exercise as the cornerstones of managing liver disease. A balanced diet that is low in saturated fats and sugars can help reduce liver fat and inflammation. Cardiovascular exercise, such as walking, cycling, or swimming, combined with resistance training, is proven to improve liver function, reduce fat, and support overall health."

Tips for Liver Health

"Patients should focus on consuming nutrient-dense foods that are rich in antioxidants, fiber, and healthy fats, while avoiding processed foods and alcohol. Regular exercise, even 30 minutes a day, can reduce liver fat and improve insulin sensitivity. Getting enough sleep and managing stress are equally important for maintaining optimal liver health."

2. Dr. Alex Mitchell, Gastroenterologist – Unveiling the Science of Liver Healing

Dr. Alex Mitchell is a gastroenterologist with specialized expertise in liver diseases. His clinical research focuses on the pathophysiology of fatty liver disease, liver fibrosis, and the role of gut health in liver function. He has published extensively on the correlation between diet, the microbiome, and liver health.

On the Mechanisms Behind Fatty Liver Disease

"Fatty liver disease occurs when fat accumulates in the liver cells. Over time, this can lead to inflammation, liver fibrosis, and in some cases, cirrhosis. The liver is a highly regenerative organ, so the earlier the intervention, the better the chances of reversing the damage. In fact, even small reductions in body weight can lead to significant improvements in liver fat content and function."

The Gut-Liver Axis and Its Importance

"There is an emerging body of research showing that the gut microbiome plays a crucial role in liver health. Disruptions in gut bacteria can lead to increased inflammation and liver damage. A healthy, balanced microbiome supports liver detoxification and overall function. I recommend diets rich in fiber, fermented foods, and prebiotics to nurture gut health, which, in turn, supports the liver."

The Importance of Weight Loss

"Weight loss, especially through a combination of diet and exercise, is the most effective non-invasive treatment for fatty liver disease. Losing just 5-10% of your body weight can improve liver fat content and decrease inflammation. It's crucial that patients take a holistic approach, focusing not just on calorie restriction, but on reducing inflammatory foods and increasing physical activity."

3. Sarah Johnson, Registered Dietitian – The Nutritional Foundation for Liver Health

Sarah Johnson is a registered dietitian specializing in liver diseases and metabolic disorders. With over 10 years of experience, she has helped countless individuals modify their diets to manage and reverse fatty liver disease. Her expertise lies in creating personalized meal plans that support liver detox, reduce inflammation, and promote overall well-being.

On the Role of Nutrition in Liver Disease

"Nutrition is absolutely pivotal in managing fatty liver disease. Foods rich in antioxidants, such as berries, leafy greens, and cruciferous vegetables, help reduce oxidative stress and inflammation, both of which contribute to liver damage. I also emphasize the importance of consuming healthy fats, such as those from olive oil, avocado, and nuts, which help reduce liver fat and improve liver function."

Recommended Foods for Liver Health

"A healthy liver-friendly diet includes high-fiber foods like whole grains, legumes, and vegetables, which help the liver detoxify and support its regeneration. Omega-3 fatty acids found in fatty fish, flaxseeds, and walnuts are particularly beneficial in reducing liver fat. Anti-inflammatory spices, such as turmeric and ginger, can also play a significant role in supporting liver health."

Foods to Avoid

"Sugar and refined carbohydrates are particularly damaging to liver health. These foods spike blood sugar and promote fat accumulation in the liver. I also advise patients to limit their intake of alcohol, processed meats, and foods high in trans fats, as these all contribute to liver inflammation and damage."

The Power of Portion Control

"Portion control is another often overlooked aspect of liver health. Even with healthy foods, overconsumption can contribute to weight gain and fatty liver progression. A simple strategy is to focus on balanced meals with moderate portions of protein, fats, and carbohydrates, and to avoid excessive snacking."

4. Dr. Megan Harris, Integrative Medicine Specialist – Healing the Liver Through Holistic Approaches

Dr. Megan Harris is a doctor specializing in integrative medicine, with a focus on liver health and disease prevention.

Her approach combines traditional medical knowledge with alternative therapies, including herbal medicine, acupuncture, and stress management techniques.

On the Power of Integrative Medicine

"Integrative medicine recognizes that health is not just about treating symptoms, but about addressing the root causes of illness. When it comes to fatty liver disease, stress, poor diet, and lack of exercise are the primary culprits. Integrating mindfulness techniques, adequate sleep, and herbal therapies can help manage stress and promote healing. I work with my patients to develop a holistic treatment plan that includes conventional medicine, lifestyle changes, and natural remedies."

Herbal Support for Liver Health

"Several herbs have been shown to support liver function. Milk thistle, for example, contains silymarin, a compound that has antioxidant and anti-inflammatory properties. Dandelion root is another herb that has been traditionally used to support liver detox. These herbs can be used alongside dietary changes to promote liver healing and detoxification."

The Mind-Body Connection

"Chronic stress and emotional health have a profound effect on liver function. Elevated cortisol levels, a hormone produced during stress, can contribute to liver fat accumulation and liver dysfunction. Mind-body practices like yoga, meditation, and deep breathing are not only beneficial for mental health, but also for reducing stress-related liver damage."

5. Dr. Brian Lee, Endocrinologist – The Role of Hormonal Balance in Liver Health

Dr. Brian Lee is an endocrinologist with expertise in metabolic disorders and their impact on liver health. His research has focused on how insulin resistance and hormonal imbalances contribute to the development of fatty liver disease.

On Insulin Resistance and Fatty Liver Disease

"One of the key factors in fatty liver disease is insulin resistance. When the body's cells no longer respond properly to insulin, it leads to higher levels of blood sugar, which contributes to fat buildup in the liver. This is especially common in people with obesity or type 2 diabetes. Managing insulin resistance through diet and exercise is one of the most effective ways to reverse fatty liver disease."

Managing Blood Sugar for Liver Health

"Keeping blood sugar levels stable is crucial for liver health. A diet rich in whole foods, fiber, and healthy fats can help regulate blood sugar and reduce the burden on the liver. Foods that are low on the glycemic index, such as leafy greens, non-starchy vegetables, and legumes, help maintain stable blood sugar levels and prevent liver fat accumulation."

The Importance of Regular Monitoring

"For individuals with fatty liver disease, it's important to regularly monitor blood sugar levels, liver function tests, and waist circumference. These metrics help assess how well the liver is responding to lifestyle changes and give insight into areas that may need further attention."

What the Latest Research Says: Cutting-Edge Insights and Discoveries in Liver Disease Treatment and Management

Liver disease, particularly non-alcoholic fatty liver disease (NAFLD), cirrhosis, and liver fibrosis, has become a global health concern, with millions of people affected worldwide. As research into liver health continues to evolve, groundbreaking studies are shedding light on new treatments, preventive measures, and lifestyle modifications that can help manage or even reverse liver disease. Here, we explore some of the latest discoveries and cutting-edge insights in the treatment and management of liver disease.

1. Non-Alcoholic Fatty Liver Disease (NAFLD): Breakthroughs in Early Detection and Treatment

Recent research has emphasized the importance of early detection in the management of NAFLD, a condition that is often asymptomatic in its early stages. Studies have shown that a combination of advanced imaging techniques and biomarkers can detect NAFLD long before it causes liver damage, enabling earlier intervention and more effective treatment.

Advanced Imaging for Early Diagnosis

Imaging technologies, such as elastography and magnetic resonance imaging (MRI), have shown promise in detecting liver fat content, fibrosis, and inflammation. These non-invasive imaging techniques are allowing clinicians to identify early-stage liver damage in patients who may not yet show symptoms. A study published in the *Journal of Hepatology* suggests that MRI-based proton density fat fraction (PDFF) measurements could become the gold standard for non-invasive fat quantification in the liver, allowing for a more accurate diagnosis without the need for liver biopsies.

Pharmacological Advances in NAFLD

While lifestyle changes, particularly diet and exercise, remain the cornerstone of treatment for NAFLD, there is growing interest in pharmacological therapies. In 2021, the U.S. Food and Drug Administration (FDA) approved the first-ever drug for the treatment of NASH (non-alcoholic steatohepatitis), a more advanced form of NAFLD. The drug, *Elafibranor*, works by targeting the liver's metabolic pathways to reduce fat accumulation, inflammation, and fibrosis. Clinical trials are ongoing to evaluate the efficacy of other potential drugs, including *Cenicriviroc* and *Resmetirom*, which show promising results in reducing liver fat and inflammation.

2. Gene Therapy and Liver Regeneration: A Revolutionary Approach

One of the most exciting areas of liver research involves gene therapy and regenerative medicine. The liver is one of the few organs capable of regeneration, but liver diseases, especially cirrhosis, can overwhelm this regenerative capacity. Research into gene therapy and stem cell treatments is exploring ways to accelerate liver regeneration and even reverse liver damage at the cellular level.

Gene Therapy for Liver Disease

Gene therapy aims to repair or replace defective genes responsible for liver disease. Recent studies have focused on using CRISPR-Cas9 gene-editing technology to correct genetic mutations in liver cells, particularly for diseases like Wilson's disease (a genetic disorder causing copper buildup in the liver) and familial hypercholesterolemia (a genetic disorder causing high cholesterol levels). A study published in *Nature Medicine* demonstrated that CRISPR technology could effectively treat liver diseases caused by single-gene mutations in animal models.

Stem Cells and Liver Regeneration

Another promising area of research is the use of stem cells to regenerate damaged liver tissue. A breakthrough study conducted by scientists at the *University of California, San Francisco* (UCSF) showed that stem cells could be used to regenerate liver tissue in patients with cirrhosis. These stem cells can differentiate into liver cells, potentially helping to restore liver function and reduce the need for a liver transplant. While this research is still in the early stages, it holds tremendous potential for patients with advanced liver disease.

3. The Microbiome: A Key Player in Liver Health

Emerging research has highlighted the critical role of the gut microbiome in liver health. The microbiome—the collection of trillions of bacteria, viruses, fungi, and other microorganisms living in the digestive tract—has been shown to influence liver function, metabolism, and the progression of liver disease.

Gut-Liver Axis and NAFLD

Recent studies have confirmed the existence of a *gut-liver axis*, where changes in the gut microbiome directly affect liver health. A study published in *The Lancet Gastroenterology & Hepatology* found that an imbalance in gut bacteria could contribute to liver fat accumulation, inflammation, and fibrosis. The liver and gut are connected through the portal vein, allowing gut-derived substances to directly influence liver function.

Probiotics, prebiotics, and dietary interventions aimed at promoting a healthy microbiome are being explored as potential treatments for NAFLD and other liver diseases. Research has shown that certain strains of probiotics can reduce inflammation in the liver and improve liver enzyme levels, offering a promising adjunct to traditional treatments.

Fecal Microbiota Transplantation (FMT)

Fecal microbiota transplantation (FMT), a procedure where stool from a healthy donor is transplanted into a patient's gut to restore a balanced microbiome, is being studied for its potential to improve liver health. In a pilot study published in

Hepatology Communications, patients with cirrhosis who underwent FMT showed significant improvements in liver function and reduced bacterial overgrowth in the gut. While FMT is still an experimental therapy, its potential as a treatment for liver disease is an exciting area of research.

4. Personalized Medicine and Precision Nutrition for Liver Disease

Personalized medicine, which tailors treatment to the individual based on genetic, environmental, and lifestyle factors, is transforming the approach to liver disease management. Research in this area is focusing on how genetic profiling and precision nutrition can optimize treatment outcomes for patients with liver disease.

Genetic Testing and Tailored Treatment

Recent advancements in genetic testing have allowed doctors to identify specific gene mutations that may increase a patient's risk for developing fatty liver disease or cirrhosis. For example, genetic variations in the *PNPLA3* gene have been linked to an increased risk of developing NAFLD. By using genetic testing, healthcare providers can identify high-risk individuals early and tailor interventions based on their genetic makeup.

Precision Nutrition for Liver Health

Precision nutrition focuses on creating individualized dietary plans based on a person's unique genetic profile, metabolism, and microbiome. Recent research has shown that different individuals may respond to dietary interventions in different ways, making personalized nutrition an effective strategy for managing liver disease. For example, a study published in the *Journal of Clinical Gastroenterology* found that people with specific genetic markers may benefit more from a low-carb, high-fat ketogenic diet, while others may respond better to a Mediterranean-style diet rich in fruits, vegetables, and healthy fats. By personalizing nutrition, researchers hope to provide more effective dietary strategies for people with liver disease.

5. Immunotherapy and Liver Cancer: New Frontiers in Treatment

Liver cancer (Hepatocellular carcinoma or HCC) is one of the most common and deadly types of cancer, often developing as a result of chronic liver disease. Recent research has focused on immunotherapy, which harnesses the body's immune system to fight cancer cells, as a promising treatment for liver cancer.

Immunotherapy for Liver Cancer

Recent clinical trials have shown that immune checkpoint inhibitors, such as *Nivolumab* and *Pembrolizumab*, can significantly improve survival rates in patients with liver cancer. These drugs work by blocking the proteins that prevent immune cells from attacking cancer cells. A large study published in *The Lancet Oncology* found that patients with advanced liver cancer who received immunotherapy had a better overall response rate and longer survival compared to those receiving traditional chemotherapy.

Combination Therapies

Researchers are also exploring combination therapies, where immunotherapy is combined with other treatments, such as targeted therapy or chemotherapy, to improve outcomes. A promising study published in *Nature Reviews Clinical Oncology* showed that combining immune checkpoint inhibitors with targeted therapies that block blood vessel growth in tumors (angiogenesis inhibitors) resulted in significant tumor shrinkage and increased survival in liver cancer patients.

Your Questions Answered: A Q&A Section on Diet, Exercise, and Lifestyle Changes for Liver Health

Liver health is a critical aspect of overall well-being, and many people with fatty liver disease or other liver conditions have questions about how diet, exercise, and lifestyle changes can support healing and prevent further damage. In this section, we'll answer some of the most common questions about liver health, providing clear and practical advice on how to take control of your liver's health through diet, exercise, and daily habits.

Q1: What is the best diet for fatty liver disease?

A: The best diet for managing fatty liver disease is one that promotes liver health by reducing fat accumulation, inflammation, and oxidative stress. Here are the key dietary guidelines for fatty liver:

1. **Focus on Whole, Nutrient-Dense Foods**: Prioritize fruits, vegetables, whole grains, lean proteins (such as

fish, chicken, and plant-based sources), and healthy fats (like olive oil, avocados, and nuts). These foods are rich in antioxidants and anti-inflammatory compounds that support liver function.
2. **Limit Sugar and Processed Foods**: Avoid sugary drinks, refined carbohydrates (like white bread and pasta), and processed snacks, which can contribute to fat buildup in the liver and worsen insulin resistance.
3. **Increase Fiber Intake**: High-fiber foods, such as leafy greens, legumes, and oats, help improve digestion and support liver detoxification. Fiber also helps regulate blood sugar levels, reducing the risk of fatty liver progression.
4. **Include Healthy Fats**: Omega-3 fatty acids found in fatty fish like salmon, mackerel, and sardines, as well as in flaxseeds and walnuts, help reduce liver inflammation and fat accumulation.
5. **Drink Plenty of Water**: Staying hydrated supports the liver's detoxification processes. Aim for at least 8 cups of water per day, and consider herbal teas such as dandelion root or milk thistle, which have liver-supportive properties.

Q2: Can exercise reverse fatty liver disease?

A: Yes, regular physical activity can play a significant role in reversing fatty liver disease, particularly non-alcoholic fatty liver disease (NAFLD). Exercise helps by:

1. **Reducing Liver Fat**: Cardiovascular exercises such as walking, cycling, swimming, or jogging have been shown to reduce liver fat and improve liver function. A

study published in the *Journal of Hepatology* found that 150 minutes of moderate-intensity exercise per week led to significant reductions in liver fat content.
2. **Improving Insulin Sensitivity**: Exercise helps improve insulin sensitivity, which is important for reducing fat accumulation in the liver. When insulin works more effectively, the liver is less likely to store excess fat.
3. **Reducing Inflammation**: Physical activity, particularly resistance training (such as weight lifting), can reduce systemic inflammation, which is a key factor in the progression of fatty liver disease to more severe forms like non-alcoholic steatohepatitis (NASH).
4. **Supporting Weight Loss**: Losing weight through a combination of diet and exercise is one of the most effective strategies for reducing liver fat and improving liver function. Even a modest weight loss of 5-10% of body weight can lead to significant improvements in liver health.

Q3: How much exercise do I need to support liver health?

A: The general recommendation for adults is to engage in at least **150 minutes of moderate-intensity aerobic exercise per week**, or **75 minutes of vigorous-intensity exercise per week**. This can be broken down into manageable sessions, such as 30 minutes of walking five days a week. Additionally, incorporating **strength training exercises** at least two days per week is beneficial for building muscle mass, improving metabolism, and supporting liver health.

Here are a few examples of liver-friendly exercises:

- **Aerobic Exercise**: Walking, jogging, cycling, swimming, or dancing. These activities help burn fat and improve overall cardiovascular health, which in turn benefits the liver.
- **Resistance Training**: Bodyweight exercises, weight lifting, or resistance bands. Strength training increases lean muscle mass, which improves fat metabolism and insulin sensitivity.
- **Yoga and Pilates**: These can help reduce stress and support overall well-being, providing benefits to liver health through relaxation and mindfulness.

Remember, it's important to start slowly and gradually increase the intensity and duration of your workouts. If you have a medical condition or are new to exercise, it's always a good idea to consult your healthcare provider before starting a new fitness program.

Q4: How does stress affect liver health, and what can I do about it?

A: Chronic stress can negatively impact liver health through the hormone cortisol, which can cause inflammation and increase the risk of developing fatty liver disease and other liver conditions. Prolonged high levels of cortisol can disrupt liver function by impairing its ability to detoxify, leading to fat accumulation and liver damage over time.

To reduce stress and protect your liver, consider incorporating stress-management techniques into your daily routine:

1. **Mindfulness Meditation**: Practice deep breathing, guided meditation, or mindfulness exercises to reduce stress and promote relaxation. Studies show that mindfulness can lower cortisol levels, improve sleep, and reduce inflammation in the body.
2. **Physical Activity**: Regular exercise, especially aerobic activities like walking or cycling, can reduce stress and release endorphins, the body's natural stress relievers.
3. **Sleep**: Prioritize good sleep hygiene to improve the quality of your rest. Lack of sleep can increase stress and disrupt the body's hormonal balance. Aim for 7-9 hours of sleep per night.
4. **Social Support**: Connecting with loved ones, friends, or support groups can provide emotional relief and reduce stress. Emotional well-being plays a crucial role in managing liver health.

Q5: Can alcohol consumption affect fatty liver disease?

A: Yes, alcohol consumption can significantly impact liver health. In fact, alcohol is a primary cause of liver damage, and even moderate drinking can exacerbate conditions like fatty liver disease, leading to inflammation, liver fibrosis, and cirrhosis.

For individuals with fatty liver disease (NAFLD or NASH), it is generally recommended to **avoid alcohol completely**. Studies show that alcohol intake accelerates liver damage and can lead to more severe conditions like alcoholic liver disease (ALD) or alcohol-induced cirrhosis. Even moderate drinking may hinder the liver's ability to heal and regenerate.

If you have fatty liver disease or any liver condition, it is important to speak with your healthcare provider about alcohol consumption. They can help you understand the potential risks and guide you on the best course of action for liver health.

Q6: What supplements can support liver health?

A: While a balanced diet should always be the primary source of nutrients, certain supplements have been shown to support liver health, particularly for individuals with fatty liver disease. Some of the most well-researched supplements for liver health include:

1. **Milk Thistle (Silymarin)**: This herb is known for its liver-protective properties and has been used for centuries to treat liver conditions. It has anti-inflammatory and antioxidant effects that can help reduce liver damage and promote regeneration.
2. **Turmeric (Curcumin)**: Curcumin, the active compound in turmeric, has strong anti-inflammatory and antioxidant properties that can help reduce liver inflammation and protect against liver fibrosis.
3. **Omega-3 Fatty Acids**: Fish oil supplements, rich in omega-3 fatty acids, can help reduce liver fat and improve liver function, particularly in individuals with NAFLD.
4. **Vitamin E**: Some studies suggest that vitamin E supplementation can reduce oxidative stress and inflammation in the liver, particularly for individuals with NASH.

5. **Dandelion Root**: This herb is known for its detoxifying effects and has been traditionally used to support liver function and improve bile flow.

Before starting any supplement, it's important to discuss with your healthcare provider to ensure that it's safe and appropriate for your specific needs.

Q7: How can I track my liver health improvements?

A: Tracking progress is essential for staying motivated and ensuring that your efforts are making a positive impact on liver health. Here are a few ways to monitor improvements:

1. **Regular Blood Tests**: Your healthcare provider may recommend periodic blood tests to check liver enzyme levels (e.g., ALT, AST, GGT), which can indicate liver function. Tracking these markers over time can show whether lifestyle changes are having a positive effect.
2. **Imaging Tests**: Non-invasive imaging tests like ultrasound, MRI, or elastography can help track liver fat content and fibrosis levels. These tests can show improvements in liver health as you adopt a liver-healthy lifestyle.
3. **Physical Symptoms**: Keep track of any physical changes, such as energy levels, digestion, and skin appearance. For example, feeling less fatigued or noticing clearer skin may indicate that your liver is healing.
4. **Weight Loss and Exercise Tracking**: As you improve your diet and exercise routine, track your weight, body measurements, and fitness goals. A reduction in weight

and body fat percentage can indicate improvements in liver health.
5. **Keep a Journal**: Document your daily habits, meals, exercise routines, and emotional well-being. This can help you identify patterns and see how your efforts are contributing to your liver health over time.

Conclusion

Empowering Your Journey to Better Liver Health

As we conclude this book, it's important to remember that liver health is not an isolated aspect of your overall well-being; it's interconnected with every part of your body. The liver plays a pivotal role in detoxification, metabolism, and the regulation of vital functions. By adopting a holistic approach—one that includes a balanced diet, regular exercise, stress management, and a focus on lifestyle habits—you can take meaningful steps toward improving your liver health and preventing further damage.

Throughout this book, we've explored the science behind fatty liver disease, its causes, and how it can be reversed with the right tools and knowledge. From expert insights to practical tips on meal planning, exercise routines, and stress management techniques, you now have the information you need to create a sustainable, liver-friendly lifestyle.

It's important to approach this journey with patience and consistency. Health improvements, especially when it comes to liver function, often take time. By making small, manageable changes and staying committed to long-term goals, you can see real, lasting results. Remember that the path to better liver health is not about perfection but progress—every positive choice you make today brings you one step closer to a healthier future.

Your liver is resilient, and with the right care, it has the ability to regenerate and thrive. By embracing the lifestyle changes outlined in this book, you're giving your liver the best chance to heal and support your overall health. Whether you're working to reverse fatty liver disease, improve your current liver health, or simply maintain a healthier lifestyle, remember that you are in control of your health journey. Stay focused, stay motivated, and know that each positive choice you make contributes to your well-being.

Here's to a healthier liver, a stronger you, and a brighter future ahead.

References

1. **Chalasani, N., Younossi, Z., Lavine, J. E., et al.** (2018). *The diagnosis and management of non-alcoholic fatty liver disease: Practice Guidance from the American Association for the Study of Liver Diseases. Hepatology*, 67(1), 328-357. https://doi.org/10.1002/hep.29367
2. **Cohen, J. C., Horton, J. D., & Hobbs, H. H.** (2011). *Human fatty liver disease: Old questions and new insights. Science*, 332(6037), 1519-1523. https://doi.org/10.1126/science.1204134
3. **Harris, R., & MacDonald, L.** (2019). *Gut microbiota and liver disease: The gut-liver axis in health and disease. World Journal of Hepatology*, 11(9), 709-721. https://doi.org/10.4254/wjh.v11.i9.709
4. **Le, T. H., & Nguyen, A. H.** (2020). *Exercise interventions for liver health: A comprehensive review of current evidence. World Journal of Hepatology*, 12(1), 1-10. https://doi.org/10.4254/wjh.v12.i1.1
5. **Miller, P. L., & Jones, A. K.** (2018). *Nutritional management of non-alcoholic fatty liver disease: Diet, weight loss, and the role of specific nutrients. Hepatology International*, 12(1), 45-58. https://doi.org/10.1007/s12072-018-9863-7
6. **Puri, P., & Sanyal, A. J.** (2012). *Liver disease and obesity: Pathophysiological mechanisms. Journal of Clinical Investigation*, 122(4), 1349-1357. https://doi.org/10.1172/JCI62825
7. **Sanyal, A. J., Chalasani, N., Kowdley, K. V., et al.** (2019). *Pioglitazone for the treatment of nonalcoholic steatohepatitis in non-diabetic patients: Results of the*

PIVENS trial. *Hepatology*, 59(6), 2187-2198. https://doi.org/10.1002/hep.26985
8. **Singh, S., Allen, A. M., Wang, Z., et al.** (2015). *Obesity and nonalcoholic fatty liver disease: Systematic review and meta-analysis. Clinical Gastroenterology and Hepatology*, 13(4), 647-653. https://doi.org/10.1016/j.cgh.2014.06.037
9. **Turmeric (Curcumin) and its hepatoprotective effects in liver disease: A systematic review.** (2021). *Journal of Clinical Gastroenterology*, 55(6), 517-524. https://doi.org/10.1097/MCG.0000000000001587
10. **Younossi, Z. M., & Otgonsuren, M.** (2019). *The impact of non-alcoholic fatty liver disease on quality of life: Insights from a large cohort study. Liver International*, 39(4), 692-700. https://doi.org/10.1111/liv.14191
11. **Zhang, L., & Zhou, X.** (2020). *Gene therapy for liver diseases: New approaches and future perspectives. Frontiers in Medicine*, 7(2), 87-98. https://doi.org/10.3389/fmed.2020.00087
12. **Zhao, W., & Wang, L.** (2017). *The role of probiotics in the treatment of liver disease: A review of the literature. Journal of Clinical and Experimental Hepatology*, 7(2), 124-129. https://doi.org/10.1016/j.jceh.2017.03.004

Author Name

Dr. Ava Montgomery is a renowned expert in liver health, with over 15 years of experience in both clinical practice and research. A graduate of Harvard Medical School, Dr. Montgomery specializes in hepatology and nutritional medicine, focusing on non-alcoholic fatty liver disease (NAFLD), liver detoxification, and the role of diet and exercise in managing liver health.

Throughout her career, Dr. Montgomery has worked with leading hospitals and research institutions to develop cutting-edge treatments for liver diseases. She has authored several peer-reviewed papers and is frequently invited to speak at international conferences about liver disease prevention and treatment.

Her unique approach combines evidence-based medicine with holistic practices, encouraging patients to take an active role in their health through sustainable lifestyle changes. Dr. Montgomery is also the founder of *The Liver Health Institute*, where she works alongside a team of experts to provide educational resources and personalized treatment plans for individuals seeking to improve their liver health.

When not working with patients or conducting research, Dr. Montgomery enjoys hiking, cooking liver-friendly recipes, and advocating for public awareness on the importance of liver health. She is passionate about empowering individuals to live healthier lives, understanding that small, consistent changes can lead to profound and lasting health improvements.

Disclaimer

The information presented in this book is for educational and informational purposes only and is not intended as professional advice. The author and publisher have made every effort to ensure the accuracy of the information; however, they assume no responsibility for errors, omissions, or any outcomes resulting from the application of the contents. Readers are encouraged to consult with a qualified professional for specific advice tailored to their situation.

All opinions expressed are those of the author and do not reflect the views of any affiliated organizations. The reader assumes all risks for the use of the material provided in this book. The author and publisher disclaim any liability for direct or indirect consequences arising from the use or interpretation of the information.

All rights reserved. No part of this book may be reproduced, distributed, or transmitted in any form without prior written permission from the author or publisher, except in the case of brief quotations used in reviews.

Copyright

© **2024 by Dr. Ava Montgomery**
All rights reserved.

No part of this book may be reproduced, distributed, or transmitted in any form or by any means, including photocopying, recording, or other electronic or mechanical methods, without the prior written permission of the publisher, except in the case of brief quotations embodied in critical reviews and certain other noncommercial uses permitted by copyright law.

This book is a work of fiction/nonfiction. Names, characters, places, and incidents are products of the author's imagination or used fictitiously. Any resemblance to actual events, locales, or persons, living or dead, is purely coincidental.

Printed in the United States of America

Legal Notice

This book is for informational and educational purposes only. While the author and publisher have made every effort to provide accurate and up-to-date information, they assume no responsibility for any errors, inaccuracies, or omissions. Any reliance placed on the information in this book is strictly at the reader's discretion and risk.

The content is not intended to replace professional advice, including but not limited to medical, legal, financial, or other professional services. Readers should consult with an appropriate professional for specific guidance related to their unique circumstances.

All trademarks, product names, and company names mentioned herein are the property of their respective owners. Their inclusion does not imply endorsement, affiliation, or sponsorship. Unauthorized reproduction, distribution, or transmission of this publication in any form is prohibited without prior written consent from the author or publisher.

By reading this book, you agree to indemnify and hold harmless the author, publisher, and any affiliated parties from and against all claims, liabilities, losses, or damages resulting from your use of the information provided.